# Springer Series on PSYCHIATRY

**Carl Eisdorfer, PhD, MD,** Series Editor

**Robert Paul Liberman, MD**, is Professor of Psychiatry at UCLA School of Medicine. Since 1977 he has directed the NIMH-funded Clinical Research Center, a conceptualization of schizophrenia that includes stress, vulnerability, and protective factors. Dr. Liberman has guided a group of interdisciplinary scientist–practitioners in their study of the psychobiological, pharmacological, familial, and behavioral factors that are related to the etiology, course, and treatment of schizophrenia.

With his clinical research colleagues, Liberman has developed innovative methods that have been documented to improve the functioning and quality of life of persons with serious and disabling long-term mental illness. These include behavioral family management that involves patients and their relatives in an educational process that equips them with coping, communication, and problem-solving skills, and an array of psychoeducational modules for teaching community living skills to mentally disabled persons. Several of the modules have been translated into French, German, Japanese and other languages. Dr. Liberman has written over 250 articles and 8 books. Among his awards are the Silvano Arieti Award in Schizophrenia from the American Academy of Psychoanalysis, the Samuel Hibbs Award from the American Psychiatric Association (APA) for innovations in the treatment of chronic mental illness, the APA Van Ameringen Award for Psychiatric Rehabilitation, a fellowship from the International Exchange of Experts in Rehabilitation, and the Arthur Noyes Award for Schizophrenia Research.

**Joel Yager, MD**, is Professor of Psychiatry at the UCLA School of Medicine, Director of Residency Education at the UCLA Neuropsychiatric Institute and West Los Angeles Veterans Administration Medical Center (Brentwood Division), and Associate Chief of Staff for Residency Education at Brentwood. He is also Chief of the Adult Eating Disorders Program at the UCLA Neuropsychiatric Institute.

A native of New York City, Dr. Yager graduated from the College of the City of New York and the Albert Einstein College of Medicine, and completed an internship in medicine and residency in psychiatry at the Bronx Municipal Medical Center–Albert Einstein College of Medicine. His past positions include Major in the U.S. Army Medical Corps, Fort Ord, CA, and Assistant Professor of Psychiatry at the University of California, San Diego, where he was Chief of Ambulatory Services at the University Clinic and Chief of Consultation-Liaison Services at the San Diego VA Medical Center. He has been on the faculty of UCLA since 1973.

Dr. Yager has edited three books and published more than 150 scientific papers, book chapters, and reviews in the areas of psychiatric education, eating disorders, stress and coping, and other fields of general psychiatry. He is on the editorial board of five medical journals, including the *Archives of General Psychiatry*, the *Journal of Psychiatric Education*, and the *International Journal of Eating Disorders*.

# *S*tress *in* Psychiatric Disorders

## Robert Paul Liberman, MD
## Joel Yager, MD

Editors

<br>

Springer Publishing Company
New York

Springer Publishing Company, Inc.
536 Broadway
New York, NY 10012

94 95 96 97 98 / 5 4 3 2 1

---

**Library of Congress Cataloging-in-Publication Data**

Stress in psychiatric disorders / Robert Paul Liberman, Joel Yager,
  editors.
    p.  cm.—(Springer series on psychiatry; 5)
  Includes bibliographical references and index.
  ISBN 0-8261-8310-7
  1. Mental illness—Etiology.  2. Stress (Psychology)  3. Post-
traumatic stress disorder.  I. Liberman, Robert Paul, 1937–  .
II. Yager, Joel.  III. Series.
  [DNLM: 1. Stress, Psychological—psychology.  2. Mental Disorders—
psychology.  WM 172 S915355 1994]
RC455.4.S87S776  1994
616.89′071—dc20
DNLM/DLC
for Library of Congress                                93-41244
                                                   CIP

---

Printed in the United States of America

# Contents

# Contributors

**Donald W. Bechtold, MD**, is an Assistant Professor of Psychiatry and Director of Training in Child Psychiatry at the University of Colorado School of Medicine in Denver. Dr. Bechtold attended medical school at the University of Colorado School of Medicine, and completed an internship in community medicine, a residency in general psychiatry, and a fellowship in child and adolescent psychiatry at the same institution. He has a long-standing interest in the mental health needs of American Indian and Native populations and is the recipient of an NIMH Faculty Scholar Award for studying adolescent suicide within an American Indian boarding school population.

**Patrick W. Corrigan, PsyD**, is Assistant Professor of Clinical Psychiatry at the University of Chicago, where he directs the Center for Psychiatric Rehabilitation. The Center, a joint project between the University of Chicago and the Illinois Department of Mental Health and Developmental Disabilities, develops and evaluates user-friendly, psychosocial treatments for severely mentally ill adults and their families. Dr. Corrigan has published more than 50 journal articles and book chapters in this area. He has co-edited a book with Robert Paul Liberman entitled *Behavior Therapy in Psychiatric Hospitals*.

**Calvin J. Frederick, PhD**, is an Adjunct Professor in the Department of Psychiatry and Biobehavioral Sciences at the University of California, Los Angeles, and Chief, Psychology Service, at the Department of Veterans Affairs Medical Center, West Los Angeles. Some of Dr. Frederick's previous positions include: Deputy Chief of the Center for Studies of Suicide Prevention at the National Institute of Mental Health, Chief of Research and Training Fellowships in the Center for Studies of Crime and Delinquency (later Center for Studies of Violence), and Chief of Emergency Mental Health and Disaster Assistance at the NIMH.

**Milton Greenblatt, MD**, received his Bachelor's degree from Tufts College, and his medical degree from the Tufts University School of Medicine. He has taught at the Harvard Medical School, the Boston University School of Medicine, the Tufts University School of Medicine, and the University of California, Los Angeles, where, since 1984, he has been Professor of Psychiatry, Emeritus. His professional experience also includes: Director of the Neuropsychiatric Institute Hospital and Clinics, UCLA; Executive Associate Director, Neuropsychiatric Institute, UCLA; Executive Vice Chairman and Vice Chairman, Department of Psychiatry and Biobehavioral Sciences, UCLA; and Associate Director of Psychiatry, Olive View–UCLA Medical Center. His many awards and honors include the American Psychiatric Association's Distinguished Service Award (1981).

**Sally J. MacKain, PhD**, is Assistant Professor of Psychology at the University of North Carolina at Wilmington, where she teaches and conducts research in psychosocial rehabilitation with mentally ill and mentally retarded offenders. Dr. MacKain also provides training and consultation to inpatient, outpatient, and correctional facilities throughout the United States in the development and implementation of psychosocial rehabilitation programs.

**Spero M. Manson, PhD**, is Professor, Department of Psychiatry, and Director, National Center for American Indian and Alaska Native Mental Health Research at the University of Colorado Health Sciences Center. He also serves as program codirector of the Robert Wood Johnson Foundation's Healthy Nations Initiative, an effort to assist Indian and Native communities in their struggle to reduce substance abuse. Dr. Manson received his graduate training in medical anthropology at the University of Minnesota. He publishes extensively on the assessment, epidemiology, and prevention of alcohol, drug, and mental disorders across the developmental lifespan of Indian and Native people.

**Richard H. Rahe, MD**, is Professor of Psychiatry, Department of Psychiatry and Behavioral Sciences, University of Nevada School of Medicine, Reno, where he is also Director of the Nevada Stress Center, and Medical Director of the Nevada Mental Institute. His additional current academic appointments include Professor of Psychiatry and Psychology, Uniformed Services University of the Health Sciences, Bethesda, Maryland, and Professor (Adjunct) of Psychiatry, Department of Psychiatry and the Brain Research Institute, University of California at Los Angeles.

After receiving his medical degree at the University of Washington School of Medicine, Seattle, he was awarded the McDonnel Prize for original and scholarly research in psychiatry. Dr. Rahe was co-developer, with Thomas H. Holmes, MD, of the widely known Holmes-Rahe

Stress Test. His research interests include stress and coping in several strata of human life. His research has targeted life stress and illness onset, psychosocial aspects of coronary heart disease, law-enforcement selection and training, and hostages.

Dr. Rahe retired from the U.S. Navy with the rank of captain after a 20-year tour of duty as a medical officer. His psychiatrist assignment included: member of the mental health team, Department of State, for the Americans held hostage in Iran; the Naval Support Forces, Antarctica, debriefing the winter-over personnel stationed at the South Pole; Commanding Officer, Naval Health Research Center, San Diego, and Naval Regional Medical Center, Guam.

**Robert T. Rubin, MD**, is Director of the Neurosciences Research Center at the Allegheny-Singer Research Institute and Professor of Psychiatry, Allegheny Campus of the Medical College of Pennsylvania, Pittsburgh, since May 1992. Formerly, he had been Professor of Psychiatry at the UCLA School of Medicine. Dr. Rubin is board-certified in psychiatry, and has a PhD in physiology, with an emphasis on neuroendocrinology. He has been an NIMH Research Scientist Awardee since 1972, and a Fulbright-Hays Senior Research Scholar. Dr. Rubin's research focus has been on the neuroendocrinology of affective and anxiety disorders. He has served as President of the International Society of Psychoneuroendocrinology, and was editor-in-chief of the journal *Psychoneuroendocrinology* from 1981 to 1992. His additional current research interest is in functional neuroimaging, especially single-photo emission-computed tomography.

**James H. Shore, MD**, is Professor and Chairman, Department of Psychiatry, University of Colorado Health Sciences Center, and Superintendent of the Colorado Psychiatry Hospital. He received his medical degree from Duke University, did his medical internship at the University of Utah in 1966, and completed his psychiatry residency training at the University of Washington in Seattle. His past positions include Chief of the Mental Health Office, Portland Area Indian Health Service, Director of the Community Psychiatry Training Program at the Oregon Health Sciences University, and Professor and Chairman of the Department of Psychiatry and Assistant Dean in the School of Medicine at the Oregon Health Sciences University.

Dr. Shore is a Director of the American Board of Psychiatry and Neurology, Chairman of the APA Council of Medical Education, Past-President of the American Association of the Chairmen of Departments of Psychiatry, Fellow of the American Psychiatric Association and American

College of Psychiatrists, and Chairman of the Laughlin Fellowship Committee of the American College of Psychiatrists, among others. His professional interests include psychiatric education and administration, public and transcultural psychiatry, impaired physicians, addictions, stress disorders, suicide, and depression.

**Herbert Weiner, MD**, is Professor of Psychiatry and Biobehavioral Sciences at the University of California, Los Angeles. He was educated at Harvard College and the College of Physicians and Surgeons of Columbia University. He has written numerous articles and book chapters, and has authored and/or edited 19 books. He has been a Fellow at the Center for Advanced Studies in the Behavioral Sciences, Stanford, California, and a resident-scholar at the Bellagio Center of the Rockefeller Foundation. He has received a John Simon Guggenheim Fellowship, the Commonwealth Fund Grant Award, and the Research Career Development Award. More recently he was awarded the Alexander von Humboldt Prize, and a Fulbright Fellowship.

**Louis Jolyon West, MD**, is Professor of Psychiatry at UCLA, where for 20 years he was also Chairman of the Department of Psychiatry and Biobehavioral Sciences, Director of the Neuropsychiatric Institute, and Psychiatrist-in-Chief of the Medical Center. Previously, he served as Professor and Head of the Department of Psychiatry, Neurology, and Behavioral Sciences at the University of Oklahoma. Dr. West's research has contributed to a number of areas, including substance abuse, pain, sleep, disorders of consciousness, hallucinations, hypnosis, and various other clinical psychiatric issues. His interests also have included developments in social psychiatry racism, terrorism, and violence. He has studied the process of recruitment into religious, psychotherapeutic, and political cults, as well as the physical and psychological methods used to induce compliant behaviors in captives or other dominated persons. Dr. West is the author or editor of eight books and numerous articles on these and related topics.

As an educator, Dr. West is perhaps best known for the systematic inclusion of behavioral sciences into medical education. His long list of awards and honors includes the Vestermark Award of the American Psychiatric Association and the National Institute of Mental Health for his contributions to medical and psychiatric education, and the Leo J. Ryan Award of the Cult Awareness Network.

# Foreword

This book of scholarly chapters on the subject of stress in psychiatry is dedicated to the memory of Ransom Arthur, MD, who pioneered investigations on stress during a long career as head of the U.S. Naval Neuropsychiatric Research Laboratories in San Diego. Ransom Arthur was a role model for a generation of researchers on stress and nurtured the careers of hundreds of colleagues who worked under him when he was Executive Vice Chairman of the UCLA Department of Psychiatry, Associate Dean of the UCLA School of Medicine, Dean of the University of Oregon School of Medicine, and Chief of Staff of the Brentwood Veterans Affairs Medical Center in Los Angeles.

Ransom Arthur was a man of wide interests whose curiosity and appetite for knowledge are aptly described by the famous line from one of the dramas of Terence, the Second-Century B.C. Roman poet who wrote: "I am a human being: I think nothing of what pertains to man is foreign to me." Like an illustrious physician predecessor, Thomas Hodgkin—whose universal interest in humanity included diseases of the lymph nodes, stethoscopes, slavery, geology, American Indians, and the education of London's poor—Ransom Arthur had a scholarly interest in everything that affects mankind. He was an omnivorous reader. Classics and poetry, great novels and short stories, plays, detective stories, history books and biographies, philosophy, medical and scientific journals, newspapers from London to Los Angeles, intellectual commentary, *Scientific American*, the best sports reporting—none of these escaped Ransom's sharp eyes. He always had serious and light reading in progress concurrently.

He graduated from the University of California–Berkeley and Harvard Medical School and completed specialty training in both pediatrics and psychiatry. At Berkeley he was an intercollegiate-class swimmer and continued to be an excellent swimmer for the rest of his life, despite the handicaps of an inexorable form of rheumatoid arthritis. He was greatly interested not only in reading and sports, but also in people from all walks of life. Ransom enjoyed trying to respectfully understand not only humanity in general, but also each individual he encountered. His respect and affection for others was warmly reciprocated by his family, colleagues, students, patients, teachers, and all others who knew him.

Ransom was exceptional in still another way: He was a practical man in the sense that he successfully strove to improve behavior, not simply to explain it. Thus when he served in the Navy his research elucidated severe stress, but, in addition, he devised feasible means of mitigating or preventing the adverse effects of stress. His methods have been widely emulated.

It is, therefore, altogether fitting that a large number of Ransom's colleagues and students chose stress as a topic of a farewell symposium when Ransom was obliged by his old foe, rheumatoid arthritis, to retire from the faculty of the UCLA School of Medicine. This book is a collection of papers related to stress in psychiatry, presented in Ransom Arthur's honor as a memorial to a remarkable physician, teacher, scientist, philosopher, and friend.

SHERMAN M. MELLINKOFF, M.D.
*Dean Emeritus*
*UCLA School of Medicine*

# Preface

Stress is ubiquitous in the human condition. The nature and consequences of stress permeates research and clinical work in all areas of psychiatry and the biobehavioral sciences. Investigators and clinicians alike are concerned with delineating the manifestations, understanding and determinants, assessing the effects, and devising strategies to both prevent and treat the negative consequences of stress. All levels of inquiry have been harnessed to the study of stress, from the biological, through clinical phenomena affecting individuals, to societal and cultural arenas.

The nonspecific nature of stress is translated into specific forms of psychiatric and biomedical disorders through the confluence of socioenvironmental stressors with specific vulnerabilities possessed by individuals through their biobehavioral endowments. Protective factors, found within the environment and the person, can mitigate or buffer the noxious effects of stress superimposed on vulnerability. Primary among personal protective factors are the coping capacities and competencies of individuals as they confront stressors. Thus a model of understanding the way in which stressors form the environment—whether they be psychosocial events or physiochemical substances—actually create stress in any given individual requires knowledge of the individual's vulnerabilities, coping, and competence.

This volume brings together a group of scholarly reviews that comprise "cutting edge" issues in contemporary stress research. Each of the chapter authors have conducted original research in the area of their expertise. By combining their own research findings with informed overviews of the field, the authors provide a wide range of stimulating and heuristic perspectives.

Herbert Weiner's chapter provides a thorough examination of current thinking in the psychobiology of stress. The complexities of physiological regulation in organisms are presented from the point of view of nonlinear dynamics, a perspective gaining considerable attention only within the past few years. Robert Rubin's chapter considers a large body of work, conducted mostly in Rubin's laboratory, dealing with clinical psychoendocrinology. This research demonstrates the lawfulness of endocrine-related stress responses in normal humans and patients with depressive disorders.

Robert Liberman's work on schizophrenia, the most stressful and disabling of all psychiatric disorders, has emphasized stress-induced relapse. The specific vulnerabilities of each patient can be keyed to the design or interventions for enhancing the coping skills of patients who are pummeled by a wide range of toxic influences.

Richard Rahe has been one of the most seminal researches in the field of human stress. The Holmes and Rahe Schedule of Recent Events has been used in literally thousands of research studies, and the ideas embodied by these studies have permeated American culture at large, in part through the attention given to them in Alvin Toffler's influential book, *Future Shock*, and in scores of magazine and newspaper articles. The research described in this volume depicts Rahe's recent work that integrates what has been learned from studies of combat-related stress.

Sociocultural stressors have had major adverse impacts on the lives of Native Americans. Uprooted from their traditional customs and tribal values, youthful Native Americans are prey to a wide variety of stressors—including alcohol and drug abuse—that often destroy the fabric of their lives. James Shore and his colleagues at the University of Colorado Research Center on Native Americans have sympathetically studied the plight of adolescent Native Americans to identify protective as well as stress factors in their psychosocial economy.

A more recent and highly publicized source of stress comes from cults, which attract vulnerable individuals and, by trading social support, identity, and ideology for allegiance, can transform their values and identities. Louis Jolyon West has studied brainwashing and other mediating processes in totalistic cults since early in his career as a psychiatrist when he investigated the effects of brainwashing on American soldiers who were prisoners of war during the Korean War. His wide understanding of cults—more recently infused by studies of the Symbionese Liberation Army and the Scientology movement—is brought to bear on the way in which stress can adversely affect personal development and life trajectories. West also provides an in-depth, sometimes harrowing review of the effects of interpersonal violence, including domestic violence, random violence, and state-mediated violence such as political torture. These common occurrences have profound and lasting impact on their many victims. Calvin Jeff Frederick adds a chapter on the treatment of persons suffering from stress disorders provoked by terrorism and national disasters.

The final chapter deals with stressful aspects of the medical profession itself. Milton Greenblatt, an eminent, longtime student of sociopolitics of psychiatric administration and of large organizations, and Joel Yager describe a study of transition states in leadership roles, how they affect the leaders who are changing, and the institutions they lead. They also offer solutions for individuals and institutions to facilitate these transitions, making them better for all concerned. Also considered is the contemporary medical profession and some of the sources of the increasing stress experienced by physicians in all specialties are examined. Findings are presented of research studies that examined the sources of distress in physicians' professional and personal lives, and then coping strategies are suggested based on the reports of those physicians who described the highest levels of professional and personal satisfaction with their lives. The chapter is concluded with a list of recommendations for coping, by both individual physicians and the profession as a whole, as they attempt to grapple with uncertain futures.

In summary, the chapters in this book offer both in-depth and wide-ranging explorations of some of the most salient and pertinent aspects of stress as it affects the psychiatric profession. Practitioners, students, and researchers will all find value in this collection.

R.P.L.
J. Y.

1st 3 chapters

physical
mental
social abilities
interactions

affects behaviour
in a social
context

# CHAPTER 1

# The Revolution in Stress Theory and Research

## Herbert Weiner

## INTRODUCTION

I shall begin by reviewing Hans Selye's concepts and data about stress. In so doing, I shall identify some of the fallacies that led stress research into a crisis about 15 years ago—a crisis that almost caused the search for the relevance of stress to disease onset to be abandoned. In the course of this endeavor I shall try to highlight the remarkable changes in our understanding that have occurred since, which have resulted in a beginning identification of the links between stress, physiological change, illness, and disease. We are also on the verge of reconceptualizing these associations by discarding once useful but now outworn concepts such as homeostasis.

## WHAT IS STRESS?

No agreed-upon definition of "stress" exists. As recently as 1970, Hans Selye (1970) defined it as "the non-specific response of the body to any demand made upon it" (p. 692). Missing from this definition was the observation that stressors also have behavioral and psychological, and not only bodily, consequences. For example, different animals have a variety of behavioral strategies for survival in dealing with the threat of predators. These behavioral responses must be appropriate to the threat or challenge if they are to succeed; were they random or indiscriminate (nonspecific) survival would not be assured. When the threat to survival is an infection, the appropriate response is immunological. If the threat to reproductive success is competition among males for mates, the appropriate response is to fight the rival, submit to him, or flee from him to find another mating partner.

_An organism will use the best method available to fit in order to defend itself. Adapt to its ever-changing surroundings by choosing_

Despite the fact that the credit for the concept of stress is customarily accorded to Claude Bernard, Walter B. Cannon, and Hans Selye, the principles briefly enunciated in the previous paragraph were first laid down by Charles Darwin. It is to him that we owe a complete reassessment of the relationship of the organism to its environment, incorporated in the concept of natural selection. In Darwin's view, the environment was in constant change (seasonal, climatic, chemical, geological, etc.), and/or it was continually being altered by its inhabitants. In the organism's struggle for existence, the environment is potentially dangerous due to the withdrawal of resources; to the disruption of health by infection, starvation, heat or cold; and to the threat posed by predators and competitors. Man, by virtue of his own activities—the promotion of war and torture; the pollution of the atmosphere, waters, and ground; and the invention of dangerous technologies—adds to Nature's threats and dangers.

In Darwin's formulation, the environment was challenging, dangerous, "stressful", and full of potential or actual obstacles. Only the fittest survived. Thus the question arose: how does the organism deal with these challenges and stresses, avoid danger, and overcome obstacles to survive and reproduce?

Yet the environment also contains resources, cooperative conspecifics, and shelter. It is a source of information for whose reception and processing peripheral receptors and the brain have evolved. This information is analyzed, classified, stored, checked against past stores, and synthesized by the brain, and leads to specific and appropriate actions. These actions include selection of environments by the organism in order to bring it into more favorable conditions than mere random movements would. Animals determine what aspects of the environment are relevant and which can be ignored; they sense and respond to environmental changes with coordinated physiological and behavioral patterns (Levins & Lewontin, 1985).

Thus biologists study changing *response patterns* to some *aspect* of the environment or other organisms in it (e.g., the shadow of a predator hawk; the odor, sight, or sound of a sexually mature or a dominant male). Behavioral responses (and their physiological correlates) are usually indicators of food, sexual partners, or danger; they are often short-term responses, but are subject to intense selection, because they may fail. One reason for their failure is that both individuals and species vary in their capacities to respond to a given environmental challenge—they are differently adapted.

These environmental challenges and threats to the organism which elicit response patterns may be called *stresses* or *stressors*. Although the physiological responses to stressors are, with some exceptions, similar in different species and genera (Gibbs, 1986), what varies between similar species is the interpretation of the challenging or threatening signal. As Levins and Lewontin (1985) have pointed out, "the most advantageous response to a signal does not depend on . . . [its] . . . physical form but on its value as a predictor or correlate" (p. 43). Different environments or contexts require different responses. Conversely, different environments may require the same behavioral response as long as it is likely to guarantee survival. Additionally, the very system—the brain—which interprets the environment, and upon which the organism depends for survival, must be protected from being disrupted by external or internal forces.

This digression was intended for the purpose of pointing out that the concept of stress is by no means new; in fact, it goes back to Aristotle. However, the stressors that Selye (1936) employed in his first study overwhelmed his animals: they were rendered incapable of, or were prevented from mounting a patterned response. Even under the most dire challenge, animals capable of making an avoidant response suffered less organ damage than those who were prevented from doing so (Weiss, 1971).

Furthermore, stress research has been biased by a tradition of controlled experiments in biologically irrelevant (electric shock), inappropriate (injections of croton oil), or impoverished contexts (social animals isolated in cages). Stress has been equated with anesthesia (ether stress). It was administered to highly trained animals made to perform stereotyped, biologically irrelevant tasks—except and possibly, the avoidance of pain. From such unnatural experimental conditions and the effects they produced—gastric erosions, adrenal hyperplasia, and hemorrhagic damage to the organs of the immune system—conclusions were drawn as to how animals behave in nature, how the brain "works," and how disease (organ damage) is produced.

## A Definition and Classification of Stress

The concept of stress flows naturally from Darwin's formulation of natural selection. Stresses are selective pressures that derive from the physical and social environment. They are challenging, or threatening to the survival, integrity and reproductive success of individuals and of groups. In animals, they are particularly intense at certain times during the life cycle—for example, during breeding. Breeding requires a chain of favorable or optimal environmental conditions which assure food supplies, housing of offspring, the correct temperature, conditions, and relative protection from predators (Crews & Moore, 1986).

Organisms vary in their capacity to respond to, meet, deal with, overcome, or escape from challenges and threats; those who cannot or do not fail to survive or fall ill. Therefore, it should not be surprising that individual differences in response to stress occur—a principle which we also owe to Darwin.

Thus stress can be conceived as a threat or challenge to the integrity and survival of the organism. Based on this idea and considering the case of humans, it may be possible to provide an initial and crude taxonomy of stress (Weiner, 1985) in the following manner:

1. *Natural disasters*: Earthquakes, floods, volcanic eruptions, fire, tornados, avalanches, mud slides, pestilence, infections, toxins, drought, and famine;

2. *Man made disasters*: War, technological inventions, economic disasters, vehicular accidents, hostage-taking, torture, rape, genocide, incarceration, child abuse, etc.

3. *Personal experiences*: Disruption of human relationships by bereavement, separation, or divorce; marital and family discord; migration; forced unemployment; poverty; occupational change; "paced" work; surgery, injury, illness, and disease; examinations, etc.

Each of these categories may have both general and individual consequences. Each person interprets such experiences in his/her own manner; they have personal meanings and a different impact on each person. Some find challenges or danger exciting, others shrink or flee from them. Some welcome death; others will go to any length to survive. Therefore, it is not the event or experience per se that is stressful, but how it is perceived by, and what it means, to its beholder that initiates a process that may end in its being considered stressful. Each stressor is associated with attempts to deal with it; these, in turn, may or may not be appropriate. A critical variable in the process is a person's sense of control over the experience and over his/her actions in dealing with it. Loss of control is experienced as helplessness or giving up, for example, and is regularly associated with corticosteroid secretion in man and animals (Sapolsky, 1988).

However, stress cannot be defined solely in physiological terms, as it often has in the past. As Darwin pointed out, behavior and physiology are inseparable: together they constitute an integrated, organismic response to challenge, threat, or danger. These patterned responses (including anticipatory ones) are highly discriminated and appropriate to the specific experience. But what generates behavioral (action) and physiological patterns? They are presumed to be due to complex neural and hormonal pattern generators and motor programs involving oscillatory processes.

## Stress and Homeostasis

Since Selye's time quite another definition of stress has been put forward: it is any threat to, or disturbance of homeostasis (Hinkle, 1987; Kopin, 1989; Munck, Guyre, & Holbrook, 1984). This definition of stress is again restricted to physiological responses to stress. It is as problematic as Selye's previously cited definition, and for some of the same reasons. Stress research in recent years has taught us that "threats" or "disturbances" are not equivalent; the patterned and coordinated changes in behavior and physiology in response to a stress are exquisitely attuned to each other. A patterned "disturbance" in the circulation produced by orthostasis differs from that produced by exercise or by a threatening fight between animals. (It also seems to be stretching the meaning of the concept to include orthostasis or exercise in any classification of stress.)

The concept of homeostasis has, in fact, simply outlived its usefulness. The basis of this idea—owed to Bernard and Cannon (Bernard, 1865; Cannon, 1929) was that every physiological variable maintains a steady-state equilibrium; when perturbed, physiological reactions occur to restore the steady-state. In the past two or three decades, the realization has dawned on biologists and physiologists that every critical variable goes through oscillations; no steady-state exists. The body's fundamental operating modes are oscillatory: respiration; body temperature; blood pressure; the pulse of the heart; sleep stages; chewing; food intake; menstruation; the levels of hormones, neurotransmitters, immunocytes, membrane receptors, and enzyme activity; and the cell cycle all go through regular oscillations on a number of time scales (second by second, circhoral, circadian, monthly, seasonal, etc.) (Garfinkel, 1983; Rapp, Mees, & Sparrow, 1981; Yates, 1982).

One reason for the existence of oscillations is that most, if not all, subsystems and systems of the body are arranged in and regulated by negative feedback loops. For example, the subsystem controlling ovarian secretion begins with the hypothalamic luteinizing hormone releasing hormone (LHRH) which stimulates oscillatory (pulsatile) secretion of luteinizing hormone (LH) by the anterior pituitary gland, that in turn causes estradiol ($E_2$) to be produced and secreted by the ovary. Estradiol usually inhibits LHRH secretion (Abraham, 1983; Smith, 1980). If this inhibition is sufficiently steep, the overall system will oscillate. The steepness of the inhibition may increase to critical levels at puberty because the hypothalamic (preoptic and arcuate) neurons become more "sensitive" to $E_2$. As a result, oscillation in the system begins—a bifurcation has occurred—and menarche is initiated. (Of course, the system is more complexly regulated: throughout the menstrual cycle $E_2$ and progesterone levels change, to account in part for intermittence in the menstrual cycle. Additionally, hypothalamic, catecholaminergic and peptidergic neurons regulate the secretion of LHRH and its gonadotrophin–associated peptide).

The nonlinear concept of bifurcation entails a qualitative change from one (stable) oscillatory mode to another. An example of such a transition is the midcycle LH pulse that ends with ovulation—an intermittent process which cannot be accounted for by any single-loop, oscillatory system. To complicate the matter even further, a single variable may oscillate within two separate timeframes, five to six oscillations (with a mean duration of 28 minutes) in serum cortisol occur in man during any 24-hour period. These are in turn superimposed on a circadian oscillation (also about 24 hours in length) whose nadir occurs in the first hours of the night. Of equal importance is that the adrenocorticotrophic hormone (ACTH) shows a similar circadian oscillation as cortisol. Yet, and despite its close link to episodic corticosteroid secretion, it also oscillates 10 times in a 24-hour period with each oscillation lasting about 140 minutes. In addition, oscillatory systems may appear to be closely coupled—for example, sleep and the circadian oscillation of cortisol secretion. We know, however, that these systems may be uncoupled (e.g., by sleep reversal).

Abnormal functioning (illness or disease), in this view, occurs when a system loses the stability of its usual operating mode (engineers calls this a "failure mode"). Each form of abnormal functioning can be conceived of as a bifurcation to a mode that "models the dynamical patterns of the pathology" (Garfinkel, 1983, p. R463). The mode may either revert to an earlier one, or it may take the form of an oscillatory instability—tetanic contractions, arrhythmias and dysrhythmias, and various other altered temporal patterns. To use another idiom, discontrol or disregulation has occurred.

One may, therefore, reconceptualize the effects of a stressor. The perturbations of a system produced by it do not alter the homeostatic steady-state; rather, they induce bifurcations, forcing a system into oscillatory instability, or producing a reversion to an earlier functioning mode.

On the other hand, a subsystem that had previously oscillated by virtue of its participation in a negative feedback loop may be taken out of the loop, for example, by ectopic tumors that produce peptides; pancreatic gastrinomas; lung tumors secreting ACTH; or when receptors are pre-empted by an auto-antibody that continually stimulates unregulated thy-roid hormone secretion, as in Graves' Disease (Weiner & Mayer, 1990). Yet we do not know how stressors interact with such nonoscillating sys-tems—if they do at all!

## Selye's Diseases of Adaptation

The intimate association between stress and disease was already apparent in Selye's initial paper (1936). In the next ten years he placed the burden on the glucocorticoids as the main incitors of the anatomical effects which he had produced. As many have pointed out—most recently Munck et al. (1984)—Selye seemed to have forgotten earlier observations that adrenalectomy markedly enhances the sensitivity of animals to injury and infection. But at that time, 40 years ago, it was quite unclear whether the permissive role of the corticosteroids in endowing the normal animal with some resistance to stress was due to the mineralo- or the gluco-corti-costeroids. Nonetheless, Selye believed that many diseases—hypertension, peptic ulcer, allergic, rheumatic, and collagen diseases—were the product of excessive or "adaptive" reactions in which the corticosteroids played a pathogenetic role. He demonstrated, for example, that a high-salt diet and treatment with deoxycorticosterone acetate in a nephrectomized ani-mal produced high blood pressure (BP). He called this heterogeneous group diseases of adaptation, implying that disease was the product of "abnormal" or excessive responses to stress.

There is, however, no evidence that the most common forms of hyper-tension are the product of excessive levels of mineralocorticoids (the role of salt in this disease remains enigmatic to this date). But the *coup de grace* to Selye's theory of disease was given by the demonstration that ACTH and the corticosteroids actually suppress the manifestations of allergic, rheumatic, and collagen diseases (Hench, Kendall, Slocumb, & Polley, 1949).

Furthermore, Selye's concept of the pathogenesis of disease was a linear one. But no system or subsystem of the body, as already intimated, func-tions in a linear manner; in fact, their mode is non-linear. They are ar-ranged in complex regulatory loops. Regulation is achieved by means of a multitude of messenger signals, composed of ions, neurotransmitters, hormones, electrolytes, amino-acids, peptides, proteins, carbohydrates, fatty acids, etc. Regulation occurs at cell membranes by ion channels and by specialized, specific receptors which transduce and digitize the message. Many influences modulate these channels and receptors in an autocrine, paracrine and endocrine (hormonal and at a distance) manner. Each signal follows an oscillatory mode. Disease occurs when the system has undergone a bifurcation for a number of reasons, and regulation and the communication between cells fails (Weiner & Mayer, 1990).

# THE FRONTIERS OF STRESS RESEARCH

## Specification of the Stressor

Returning to our main thesis that "stress" responses are not global, we find in Lewis' and colleagues' work (Lewis, Cannon, & Liebeskind, 1980) that intermittent electrical shock (120 shocks every 10 seconds) applied to a rat produces a naloxone-reversible analgesia. Continuous shock (120 shocks every second) produces an analgesia uninfluenced by naloxone. Presumably, the former releases opioid peptides while at the same time it suppresses natural killer (NK) cell activity *and* accelerates the death of animals injected with a mammary ascites tumor; continuous shock does not have such effects (Shavit, Lewis, Terman, Gale, & Liebeskind, 1984).

The exquisite specificity of the outcomes of these two forms of shock is further indicated by the fact that the analgesia produced by continuous shock depends mainly on spinal mechanisms (mediated by glycine and/or substance P?) whereas intermittent shock is inferred to release endorphins (being naloxone reversible). In turn, it is assumed, but not proven, that endorphins suppress NK cell activity.

Ballieux and Heijnen (1987) have shown that we must be even more specific: alpha- and beta-endorphins have different effects on immune function—the former inhibits antibody formation to ovalbumen and the latter enhances it and also modulates T-helper cell function. In Shavit et al.'s (1984) system it must still be shown that the NK cell assay is valid *in vivo*, not only *in vitro*. Furthermore, intermittent foot shock presumably releases more than the endorphins; in fact, PRL is also released. The mammary ascites tumor cells are PRL-sensitive. Bernton, Meltzer, and Holaday (1987) have presented data to suggest that tumoricidal macrophages are activated by PRL, which stimulates the release of lymphokines from T-cells. T-cells in turn contain PRL receptors.

Were it not for the important work of Aravich, Davis, Sladek, Felten, & Felten (1987), we would only be searching for the hormonal mediation of intermittent shock. These researchers have reminded us that the immune system (including bone marrow, thymus, spleen, gut, and lymph nodes) is also under neuronal control. Post-ganglionic noradrenergic fibers run between the lymph nodules in lymphatic gut tissue. They traverse the area which contains plasma, enterochromaffin, and T-cells. In addition to noradrenalin, roles have been found for serotonin, acetylcholine, and vasopressin in the regulation of these immunocompetent cells in the gut. Such cells are also mobile, and are "sent" to the spleen. The work of Aravich et al. (1987) adds another level of complexity to the process of immunoregulation. Not only do T-cells regulate ("help" or "suppress") B-cells, but lymphokines transform T-effector cells into specific cytotoxic cells, and lymphokines (such as gamma-interferon, and interleukin-2) regulate NK cell function. Local regulation of lymphocytes and plasma cells may occur directly by amine-transmitters and peptides, or indirectly by influencing (enterochromaffin) cells that secrete chemicals that influence immunologically competent cells. The latter in turn are influenced by a variety of peptides and steroid hormones and by neural discharge, both acting at a distance. Conversely, a variety of feedback loops from the immune system and its products (including interleukin-1, CRH-like peptide, tumor-necrosis factor and antibody) influence hypothalamic cells.

## The Integration of Behavior and Physiology

Ever since Darwin, we have known that challenges by predators, enemies, or conspecifics elicit a sequence of psychobiological responses in their subjects. For heuristic reasons, one may separate out these integrated responses into:

   1) An anticipatory phase (orienting, alerting or preparatory responses);

   2) A phase of response, which may either consist of diverting or fighting the adversary, ending in victory, defeat, submission, death, or flight (Cannon, 1929).

   Each phase is characterized by *integrated* behavioral and physiological responses (Darwin, 1872, 1965). We have learned (Zanchetti, Baccelli, & Mancia, 1976) just how specific these are. The cat about to fight manifests a circulatory pattern different than that seen during the actual fight. In preparation for the fight, the cat paws the air; its blood pressure (BP) does not change; its heart rate (HR) and cardiac output (CO) fluctuate; and blood flow in the mesenteric, renal, and iliac arteries is reduced. During the actual fight—especially when prolonged and intense—BP, CO, and HR increase; vasoconstriction in the renal and mesenteric arteries is intense; but dilatation of the iliac arteries occurs, so that total peripheral resistance (PR) is reduced.

Anticipatory cardiovascular responses to exercise are also seen in animals and man. They consist of increases in HR, systolic and diastolic BP, stroke volume (SV), and CO; blood flow through the skin and large muscles rises, but falls in the mesenteric bed, resulting in a decrease in PR. During anticipation, parasympathetic constraint on the circulation is reduced.

Once combat between animals is over, the defeated mouse, rat or monkey, or an animal prevented by restraint from acting or from "coping," shows an increase in BP and PR which is not averted by beta-adrenergic antagonists. Once defeated, the animal's HR remains unchanged, but adrenocorticotrophic hormones (ACTH), corticosteroid, beta-endorphin, and prolactin (PRL) levels rise, while testosterone (T) levels fall. The defeated rodent is also profoundly analgesic. Serum catecholamine levels do not change (Henry, Stephens, & Ely, 1986). Gastric erosions occur in some restrained animals after a period of time, and are prevented from occurring by vagotomy.

So far, the emphasis has been placed on some of the cardiovascular and hormonal changes which occur during the anticipatory phase. It should not be forgotten that these changes are integrated with specific behaviors. The cat about to fight assumes a posture, preparing it to spring; it claws and bites. Its pupils are dilated, and its hair stands up.

Therefore, one must ask how is this organismic reaction brought about by the brain? We have learned from Parati, Casadei, and Mancia (1989), that a cat confronted by another's attack that is not followed by a fight shows a somewhat different pattern of cardiovascular changes. The HR and CO rise, and splanchnic and resistance vessels constrict due to increased sympathetic discharge, but skeletal muscle flow increases due to *cholinergic* sympathetic activation; thus, on balance, only a minimal BP increase occurs. This pattern, Parati has pointed out (Parati, Casadei, & Mancia, 1989) differs from the classical "defense" reaction obtained in the laboratory by stimulation of the lateral hypothalamus, striae terminalis, or dorsolateral amygdala. The cardiovascular pattern is also somewhat different—i.e., iliac flow is increased—if the cat's attacker is a dog!

One of the major advances in understanding such discrete and integrated cardiovascular responses is the documentation that there are separate circuits in the brain that underlay them and their related behavioral patterns. For instance, one of the best studied circuits is that of the above mentioned "defense" reaction first described by Hess (1957). The neural circuitry subserving it passes from the dorsomedial nucleus of the amygdala, via the striae terminalis, to the lateral (perifornical) hypothalamus in the cat. In the rabbit the ventromedial, rather than the lateral, nucleus of the hypothalamus mediates the reaction (Schneiderman, 1983). From there, neural pathways pass to the central gray complex of the brain stem and the intermedio-lateral nuclei of the medulla. Rabbits and wild rodents become tonically immobile when faced with predators. This reaction is accompanied by a fall in BP and HR, mediated by a pathway which runs from the nucleus centralis of the amygdala to the lateral hypothalamus, the lateral zona incerta of the diencephalon, the parabrachial nucleus, and to preganglionic vagal cardioinhibitory motorneurons.

LeDoux (1989) has described still two more neural circuits: one which underlies the orthostatic cardiovascular response, first described by Doba and Reis (1974), and another which subserves a conditioned emotional response (CER). By pairing sound and shock LeDoux was able to produce marked increases in BP and a "freezing" reaction. He showed that the auditory cortex is not necessary for the CER, but the medial geniculate is. A neural circuit passes from the medial geniculate, to the caudate nucleus, putamen and the lateral nucleus of the amygdala, then to its central nucleus, to the lateral hypothalamus, to the gray matter of the brain stem and presumably to the intermedio-lateral nuclei of the medulla. He also showed, as Smith et al. (1980) had previously done in another nucleus system, that the integrated behavior and cardiovascular responses can be dissociated. A lesion of the hypothalamus eliminates the BP increase but preserves the behavioral "freezing" response to the CER. Whereas a lesion in the central gray complex of the brain stem produces the opposite effects on behavior and the BP. In other words, although behavior and physiology are integrated by neural circuits, they can also be dissociated.

But we do not know under what contingencies (other than lesions) such a dissociation occurs. Our ignorance on this matter is particularly evident when studying stress responses in man. Nonetheless, Curtis and Nesse (1978) have shown that when a person who suffers from simple phobias is confronted with the object that frightens him or her, there are profound, acute fear responses (e.g., screaming and the chattering of the teeth), but no changes in levels of serum cortisol, human growth hormone (HGH) and PRL. Furthermore, our knowledge of the neurotransmitters and neuromodulators of the separate neural circuits underlying integrated behavioral and cardiovascular responses is by no means worked out.

Thus one may conclude this section of the discussion by stating that the physiological responses of the organism are exquisitely related to the stressor. Furthermore, the behavior of organisms and the cardiovascular changes occurring in them when confronted with the stressor constitute an integrated whole; one does not "cause" the other. They are both under the control of identifiable circuits within the brain. They are activated in an unknown manner by the stressor (Weiner, 1972).

It is really quite remarkable that even molecular changes specific to the stressor occur at a receptor. Drugan et al. (1989) has described that when rats are group-housed, an increase in binding of the flunitrazepam ligand to the benzodiazepine receptor is seen. Footshock, however, reduces binding of the ligand to the same receptor (which regulates the passage of chloride ions into cerebral cortical and hippocampal cells). On the other hand, electric shock has no effect on the receptor, as evidenced by the absence of changes in the binding of the ligand.

## The Long-term Consequences of Acute Stress

Almost all of experimental stress research in the past 50 years has focused upon the acute effects of stress to produce (phasic) changes in bodily function and in the behavior of the organism. Three examples of the *long-range* effects of acute stressors will now be cited. Ward and Ward (1989) in elegant studies have shown that pregnant rats exposed to light and restrained during the last week of gestation produce male offspring who, when sexually mature, do not copulate or ejaculate when tested with receptive females, but prominently display the female copulatory pattern (known as lordosis behavior) to male rats. The male offspring of stressed mothers show anatomical and hormonal changes; the sexually dimorphic, hypothalamic preoptic area is smaller than in their normal counterparts. This change is correlated with the fact that the normal surge in serum T levels in male fetuses at 18 to 19 days of gestation does not occur if the mother is stressed. Such male fetuses also have reduced plasma levels of luteinizing hormone (LH), a reduction in the hypothalamic content of the aromatase that converts androgens to estrogens in the brain and of $\Delta - 3$ beta-hydroxysteroid dehydrogenase activity in Leydig cells. Of even greater interest is the fact that all of these effects on behavior and physiology can be averted by pretreatment of the dams with naloxone prior to their being stressed, but not by treating the offspring similarly after birth.

The second example of the long-term effects of stress is owed to Ackerman (1989), who in his series of studies has documented that the premature separation of rats at 15 days has profound consequences on behavior and on every bodily system so far studied. The acute consequences of separation is that these rats do not eat or drink for 48 hours, and a fall in body temperature occurs. At the same time they showed increased motor activity, grooming, and vocalization (Ackerman, 1981; Ackerman, Hofer, & Weiner, 1978; Weiner, 1982). The long-term physiological consequences of premature separation include disturbances in HR, sleep, and body temperature regulation; a marked increase of the probability of gastric erosions on restraint when the animal is between 22 and 40 days of age; in disturbances in immune function; and in the regulation of enzyme levels (ornithine decarboxylase) and growth hormone. If the separation is carried out at 20 days of age, an additional increase in serum levels of PRL occurs. The prematurely separated animals are permanently underweight, and have decreases in the catecholamine and nucleoprotein content of their brains (Schanberg, Evoniuk, & Kuhn, 1984; Stone, Bonnet, & Hofer, 1975).

A third example of the short- and long-term effects of stress is given by Kelly and Silverman (1988). Their studies carry an important message: it is necessary to study simultaneously the subacute and long-term effects of a stressor on behavior and the anatomy of specific regions of the brain. They chose an ambiguous stressor, consisting of white noise followed by random electrical shock administered 50% of the time. The initial effect was to reduce the food and water intake of their rats during the 72 hours of the experiment. Then an acoustic startle response developed in their animals, which persisted. The 72-hour exposure to this stressor causes an increase in corticotropin releasing factor (CRF)-oxytocin (OT) secreting cells in the medial parvocellular portion of the paraventricular nucleus (PVN) of the hypothalamus. But, no changes occur in such neurons in the rostral PVN. When exposure to this stressor is extended to 10 days, the absolute number and size of detectable CRF neurons increases, but only in the medial parvocellular part of the PVN.

Such studies markedly enhance our understanding of the concept of stress. Yet we will need more studies on the chronic effects of stressors and of superimposing acute stressors on chronically stressed animals, and on animals resistant to stress (as predicted by evolutionary theory). We know virtually nothing about the genetic history or physiology of stress-resistant animals. Yet one source of individual differences in response to stressors is genetic. Ackerman (1987) for example, has shown that the Ob/Ob mouse does not need to be prematurely separated to become excessively prone to gastric erosion formation; restraint alone will do. A part of this tendency can be ascribed to the fact that this fat rodent cannot maintain its body temperature when restrained.

A second source of individual differences in response to restraint is prior experience, such as the premature separation of an animal. A third factor is its age. In Ackerman's (1981) other studies restraint has different effects at different ages. Rivier (1989) has pointed out that in the first 2 or 3 weeks of the rat's life, separation, exposure to cold or to ether, or electric shock fails to release ACTH. And yet, as in the case of other immature systems, the CRF—the releasing hormone—is capable of "overriding" a tonic inhibition of ACTH production or secretion in the first 5 days of the animal's life. Because the adrenalectomy of baby rats is followed by the secretion of ACTH when they are stressed, Ackerman believes that corticosterone tonically inhibits CRF and ACTH secretion in diminishing amounts as the animal matures. Presumably, however, the inhibitory influence of corticosterone on CRF and ACTH secretion can be overridden by administered CRF.

## THE IMPETUS TO STRESS RESEARCH GIVEN BY THE DISCOVERY OF PEPTIDES

One hopes that the history of recent stress research and the new concepts that it has generated has been correctly read. Specifically, these new developments were the result of several important discoveries leading to revisions in Selye's original ideas. They are:

1) The behavioral and physiological responses of the organism to a particular stressor are very specific (not general).

2) The physiological responses to such stressors are patterned and integrated.

3) The patterns of cardiovascular stress responses are generated by discrete neuronal circuits in the brain. Hormones are also secreted in a patterned manner in response to specific stressors.

4) Autonomically mediated and hormonal patterns are regulated by a variety of peptides present both in the brain and elsewhere in the body. The CRF not only regulates the secretion of ACTH by the pituitary, but also has autonomic nervous system effects (Brown & Fisher, 1989), characteristic of the physiological changes associated with the "defense" reaction. It stimulates an increase in the plasma concentrations of E, NE, neuropeptide-Y (NPY), glucagon and glucose, and causes an increase of mean arterial pressure, HR, and CO. The increase in HR is associated with a decrease of baroreceptor reflex sensitivity. In animals resident in an

environment familiar to them, motor activity is increased. It also pro-duces a suppression of natural killer (NK) cell function (Irwin, Vale, & Britton, 1987) and suppresses gastric acid secretion, gastric motility, and pepsin secretion. It counteracts the effect of TRH on such changes in gas-tric secretory and motor function (Garrick, Veiseh, Weiner, & Taché, 1988; Taché, Goto, LeSiege, & Novin, 1983). And as Rivier and her co-workers have shown (Rivier, Rivier, & Vale, 1986), it suppresses the pulsatile release of the gonadotrophins.

Another example of the role of a peptide in producing patterned physi-ological change has been described by Porreca, Sheldon, and Burks (1989). Bombesin and its human analog (GRP), when given intraven-ously, diminish food intake, produce vasoconstriction, and increase the tone of the pyloric sphincter. When given centrally, this peptide produces an unusual behavior—hind paw scratching—and analgesia and alters body temperature depending on the ambient temperature. It increases serum E, blood glucose, and GH levels, but suppresses PRL and TRH levels. In the stomach it promotes mucus secretion, but diminishes pepsin and acid secretion. It delays gastric emptying and small bowel transit, but increases large bowel transit. It diminishes diarrhea. It promotes nonpropulsive contractions of the gut, and micturition causing the urinary bladder to contract tonically.

In addition to producing patterned physiological changes in a number of organ systems, peptides also regulate each other, and are responsive to social and physical changes in the environment. Most importantly, they integrate behavior and the physiology of the organism. Angiotensin II, for instance, not only raises BP but produces salt eating and water drink-ing in rats—a superb way of counteracting the effects of hypovolemic shock! Luteinizing hormone releasing hormone integrates lordosis behav-ior and ovulation. Neuropeptide-Y increases carbohydrate eating, and re-leases E during exercise, while also enhancing the retention of learned material in undertrained animals (Morley, 1989).

## Problems Posed by the Discovery of the Peptides

The discovery of the brain-body peptides during the past 15 years has been revolutionary. As of the present moment, approximately 80 pep-tides are known. New ones are daily being discovered. And it has been calculated that there may be as many as 1500 or more yet-to-be-discov-ered peptides present in the brain and the body! This eventual plethora of peptides will impose an enormous intellectual challenge to those trying to understand their role in normal psychobiological functioning, under conditions of stress and in the inception of disease. In part that challenge is already upon us. I shall try to highlight some of the issues that arise:

1) In view of the fact that several peptides are colocalized in the same neurone, what determines the selective release of only one of them in response to a specific stressor (Smelik, 1985)? Is this selectivity determined by one of the many regulators of their release, such as the releasing or steroid hormones and the biogenic amines (Gibbs, 1986; Kelly & Silverman, 1988; Meister & Hökfelt, 1989; Sawchenko, 1989; Smelik, Tilders, & Berkenbosch, 1989)?

2) How is it possible that an intruding rat releases only the peptide products of the intermediate lobe of the pituitary gland, while the homecage rat has an increase in ACTH secretion, given that all of these peptides derive from a common precursor molecule (Smelik, 1985)? What determines the appropriate cleavage point of the precursor, proopiomelanocortin (POMC)? Under what conditions does this occur? Or do specific contingencies and stressors only promote the release of the stored peptides via cyclic-AMP and adenylate cyclase stimulated by CRF (Reisine, 1989)? But CRF also increases POMC synthesis!

3) Is the interaction of CRF and aVP (which enhances the release of ACTH produced by CRF alone) in part determined because separate second messenger systems exist within corticotrophs (Reisine, 1989)?

4) Some peptides clearly enhance each others' activities (CRF and aVP), and others inhibit it (CRF and the endorphins; CRF and TRH; somatostatin and TRH).

To expand this thought somewhat further: we probably need to classify the facilitatory and inhibitory actions of the peptides into two types: whether they do so phasically or tonically. This statement is based on the fact that the opioid peptides phasically inhibit the sympatho-adrenal and pituitary adrenal axes in man, in conditions associated with heightened activity (such as mental arithmetic and exercise) or the cold pressor test and hypoglycemia (Bouloux & Grossman, 1989). But the opioid peptides inhibit pituitary adrenal function in a tonic manner. They constitute a counterregulatory system to the production of some hormones (CRF, ACTH), and of E in response to certain stressors. (This statement is based on the fact that naloxone potentiates E secretion elicited by them). They also tonically inhibit other peptides, such as the LHRH under conditions of weight loss in the adult, and possibly prior to puberty.

On the other hand, both Grossman (1989) and Holaday (1989) have intimated that GH and/or PRL may tonically maintain normal levels of

NK cell activity. Further credence to this belief is given by Irwin's studies (Irwin, Vale, & Britton, 1987) which show that intraventricular CRF administration suppresses NK cell function and that this suppression is averted when a sympathetic ganglionic blocking agent is administered. However, following hypophysectomy, intraventricular CRF has no such effect, nor does ganglionic blockade. Following hypophysectomy, baseline NK cell levels are reduced. Thus one might conclude that some peptides have a tonic inhibitory function on some systems, and a tonic facilitatory function on others. They tonically maintain baseline levels, upon which phasic responses and circadian variations in levels are imposed.

5) A peptide may have both tonic and phasic actions. The nerve growth factor (NGF) regulates the growth of sympathetic and sensory neurons. But it also tonically maintains the integrity of sympathetic neurons (antiserum to NGF produces a sympathectomy). NGF in turn is regulated by thyroxine and T. The content of NGF in the salivary glands in the male mouse is six times greater than in the female (Levi-Montalcini, 1987).

Usually, NGF does not appear in detectable amounts in the bloodstream, except when male mice are replaced in a colony following social isolation. The result is that they fight violently (Aloe, Alleva, Bohm, & Levi-Montalcini, 1986). It is known that injection of NGF causes an increase in the size of sympathetic neurons and the weight and size of the adrenal glands, the induction of tyrosine hydroxylase in the adrenal medulla, and the release of renin. (This experiment supplements and complements the findings of Henry and Stephens [1977]. They showed that this experimental situation [and its enzymatic consequences] terminates with male mice developing raised systolic BP, all of which were averted by castration).

6) Another major intellectual task confronting investigators of stress is to understand how a perceived stressor leads to the release of brain peptides. An important beginning to answering this question has been given by Feldman (1989) who has mapped the input circuitry to the PVN from peripheral receptors. These input circuits are in turn mediated by different neurotransmitters. For instance, hypothalamic noradrenergic neurons mediate photic, acoustic, and painful stimuli, whereas serotonergic neurons mediate sciatic and limbic stimulation; and both lead to the release of CRF from the PVN. The CRF neurons in the PVN are in turn inhibited by corticosteroids (Sawchenko, 1989). In some PVN neurons CRF and aVP are colocalized. The release of aVP from the PVN is in part regulated by atriopeptin (Saper, 1989).

However, the problem of the transduction of the experience perceived as stressful is unsolved. As mentioned previously, an organism is alerted to the presence of a friend or of a threat in the form of a predator or an enemy. A process of rapid evaluation must take place in order to determine whether the other creature is friend or foe. Recent studies in the neurophysiology of visual perception are of some help in answering this question (Altman, 1987). The cerebral cortex apparently "makes a map" of the world spread over several different cortical areas. These maps differ according to various attributes of the stimulus or "gestalt." The retina and lateral geniculate nucleus process some of the visual input. The visual cortex determines what color the object is and in which direction in space it is moving. Parietal cortical neurons are involved in processing where in the environment the perceived object is located. In the temporal cortex there are neurons that "tell" the organism what the object is. The frontal cortex acts as a "delay circuit," allowing the animal to determine whether it is one object or another. But the pathways from these various cortical areas to neurons such as those in the PVN still need to be mapped.

## DO GENERAL AS WELL AS SPECIFIC PHYSIOLOGICAL RESPONSES TO STRESSORS OCCUR?

Although it has become clear that integrated psychobiological responses are specifically attuned to the stressor, it is still not clear whether some of these responses do not generalize across all stressors. Certainly, Selye (1970) thought that the corticosteroids were secreted under all stressful conditions. And Reisine (1989) has stated that ACTH is always secreted with all stressful stimuli. In man, this generalization does not seem to hold (Curtis and Nesse, 1978). Ursin, Baade, and Levine (1978) studied recruits learning to jump with parachutes; only those who performed poorly increased their cortisol secretion. Those men to whom jumping was an enjoyable thrill responded with increased catecholamine but no cortisol secretion. (Those who quit training had no cortisol response either.)

But even if cortisol responses occur under stressful or other conditions, they may incite cortisol "resistance" (Gormley, Lowy, Reder, Hospelhorn, Antel, & Meltzer, 1985). In some patients with major depressive disorders, and most patients with anorexia nervosa, 24-hour mean serum cortisol levels are elevated. In the latter group they are in part due to high cortisol production rates. In the former group cortisol resistance is due to the fact that the cytosolic glucocorticoid receptor is translocated. Additionally, in depressed mood states, lymphocytes incorporate more thymidine when stimulated by a mitogen in the presence of dexamethasone (in the normal state dexamethasone suppresses mitogen stimulated thymidine incorporation). Thus, in certain abnormal psychological states when excessive levels of serum cortisol obtain, the resistance to the adverse effects of cortisol may be protective.

## PSYCHOBIOLOGY OF STRESS IN MAN

Our knowledge of the human physiology associated with specific stressors is extraordinarily spotty. It is generally recognized that bereavement and separation are powerful initiators of distress, particularly at certain times in the lifecycle. They have been correlated with the onset of a variety of illnesses and diseases (Weiner, 1987). But knowledge of the psychobiology is limited to a few studies. In some persons faced with loss, the excretion of 17-hydroxy-corticosteroids is elevated (Wolff, Friedman, Hofer, & Mason, 1964), pyrimidine incorporation into mitogen-stimulated lymphocytes is lowered (Schleifer, Keller, Camarino, Thornton, & Stein, 1983), NK cell function is suppressed, and the helper to suppressor T-cell ratio is lowered (Irwin & Weiner, 1987). But urinary catecholamine levels are unchanged after bereavement or separation (Jacobs, 1987).

We also know rather little about the physiological responses consequent to unemployment. One study suggests that there is a fall in high density lipoprotein (HDL) levels, thus lowering the high density to low density lipoprotein (LDL) ratio (Saxena, 1980). Serum cholesterol and uric acid levels in the blood rise (Kasl, Cobb, & Brooks, 1968). Unemployed men change their diet, drink more alcohol, and smoke more cigarettes. They are prone to violence and an increased morbidity and mortality (Farrow, 1984). Siegrist, Matschinger, and Siegrist (1989) have shown that when employment is uncertain—when workers face the threat of losing their jobs—changes in the ratio of HDL to LDL are already seen. They show an increase in time urgent (Type A) behavior. During this period, increased cardiovascular reactivity (HR and BP) to standard laboratory stressors is followed by a period of hyporeactivity to the same stressors, suggesting that adrenergic receptors become refractory with sustained stress; only a two-step model of cardiovascular responsivity could explain the findings.

Before we can go much further, much research is needed on the physiological correlates of the many stresses to which man is subjected. Until this work is done, our understanding of the relationship of stress to human disease is limited.

However, progress is being made in our knowledge of the manner in which stress incites disease in animals (Grijalva & Roland, 1989; Taché, Stephens, & Ishikawa, 1989). Grijalva (Grijalva & Roland, 1989), and others (Stephens, Ishikawa, Weiner, Norin, & Taché, 1988; Taché et al., 1989) are working on two different models of gastric erosion formation—the former produced by lateral hypothalamic lesions, and the latter by cold restraint. These two models seem to represent the extremes of a continuum. Grijalva's animals show an increase in body temperature following the lesion, and Taché's animals have a fall in body temperature during cold restraint. A fall in body temperature occurs also in the model pioneered by Ackerman (Ackerman et al., 1978). A nagging question still remains unanswered: What form of human gastric disease do these procedures model? Nonetheless, progress has been made in our understanding of the mechanisms of cold-restraint erosion formation. A falling body temperature releases TRH, and TRH is found in high concentrations in the dorso-motor nucleus of the vagus nerve. When TRH is instilled into this nucleus in comparison to other areas of the medulla, there is increased gastric motility and acid secretion (Stephens et al., 1988). When instilled into the cisterna magna TRH produces gastric erosions (Taché et al., 1989).

Garrick and I (Garrick, Veiseh, Weiner, & Taché, 1988) are working on a model of duodenal ulcer in the rat. It appears that at least three factors are necessary in producing this form of ulcer: increased gastric motility, acid secretion, and diminished bicarbonation secretion in the duodenum. The latter most likely is produced by increased adrenergic discharge. The model also is relevant to human disease because Isenberg and his co-workers (Isenberg, Selling, Hogan, & Koss, 1987) have reported that in peptic duodenal ulcer bicarbonate secretion is decreased.

Another model relevant to human disease is the adjuvant arthritis model. Recent work carried on by Mantyh et al. (1989) suggests a pathogenetic role for another peptide, substance P. The background for this work is as follows. Mantyh discovered a new efferent pathway from the spinal cord that passes through the dorsal root ganglion to the skin and joints, whose neurotransmitter is substance P. In adjuvant arthritis an increased number of substance P receptors appear in the affected joints. Lotz and his co-workers (Lotz, Carson, & Baughan, 1987) have reported that substance P releases collagenase and prostaglandin E from synovial cells. It is known that stress can modulate adjuvant arthritis, but the mechanism by which it does so is not known. Can it activate or suppress the efferent pathway subserved by substance P?

Despite these advances in knowledge of disease in animals, the relationship of stress to human disease onset is tenuous and a source of great debate. In studies by Weiner, Thaler, Reiser, & Mirsky (1957), the likelihood of stress producing duodenal ulcer was only 14% despite the fact that the experimental population was at high risk for the disease. In future studies, the role of stress to disease onset should focus on specified high-risk populations, rather than on the general population, in order to optimize the likelihood of obtaining an effect.

## STRESS AND ILLNESS

Beginning with Selye, the main thrust of stress research has been to link stress to disease. This relationship, about which Ransom Arthur (1982) has written, is an example of the xenocthonous model of disease. In this view, disease is always caused by some external agent and ends in morbid changes in anatomy. It is the traditional biomedical model that goes back many centuries. The external agents may be as varied as gods, evil spirits, injury, viruses, bacteria, or stress.

However, only recently has the likelihood been raised that stress most commonly ends in ill health (whose names are many and varied) and not only in disease.

## STRESS AND ILL HEALTH

Both traditional medicine and, until recently, psychosomatic medicine have preoccupied themselves with disease defined by alterations in the material structure of organs and cells. When no such changes occur but a patient is ill (in ill health), he is either neglected or subjected to unnecessary diagnostic or surgical procedures designed to search out the nonexistent lesion.

To put it another way, medical traditionalists consider that structural change is the only cause of illness and their only concern. Yet, a patient may have a disease and be in good health, or be ill. *Per contra*, the patient may be ill without a disease. But he/she cannot both be in ill and good health at the same time.

Most patients who seek medical care (other than at major medical centers) do not have diseases but are in ill health. Ill health constitutes a major burden to patients, their families, and society. Those in chronically ill health spend an average of 7 days a month in bed (those in normal health average only 1/2 day). The annual medical care costs of the chronically ill is nine times greater than the annual expenditure of the average U.S. citizen (Smith, Monson, & Ray, 1986a).

Persons in ill health are symptomatic and disabled. Ill health has clearly been related to stress. For example, threatened and or actual job loss is associated with a: 70% increase in illness episodes; 150% increase in medical consultations; and a 200% increase in attendance at outpatient departments (Beale & Nethercott, 1986).

The graver and the more frequent life events other than job loss are adjudged to be by patients, the longer these patients are likely to be symptomatic, absent from work, prone to disrupt their daily routine, and visit physicians (Norman, McFarlane, & Streiner, 1985). Their reasons for consultation are a large variety of symptoms referable to the cardiorespiratory, neuromuscular, and gastrointestinal systems and associated with anxiety and depression, which are often misdiagnosed (Smith, Monson, & Ray, 1986b).

These symptoms cluster into groups in an unsystematic manner. For instance, patients with a functional or an irritable bowel syndrome hyperventilate. Hyperventilators in turn complain of neuromuscular symptoms. In fact, these patients express personal distress in terms of bodily symptoms.

A more precise analysis of the symptoms leads to the conclusion that they represent physiological changes in vital biological functions—in respiratory and cardiac rhythms, food intake, digestion, elimination, reproduction, sleep rhythms, and pain modulation. Most of these functions are oscillatory; they are disturbed when their usual oscillatory mode is changed.

These vital biological functions can be disrupted by stress; in fact, such a disruption is the more usual outcome of stress than is disease. The accumulated observational evidence is that stress experienced as distress manifests itself in a gamut of bodily symptoms which express disrupted biological functions. These assertions will be supported by two of the many "functional" syndromes of ill health.

## Two Syndromes of Ill Health

1. *Hyperventilation.* In this syndrome, the ventilatory effort exceeds the body's need for oxygen, with the result that the partial pressure of carbon

dioxide ($PaCO_2$) in arterial blood falls, and respiratory alkalosis ensues. The chronic hyperventilator shows irregular (oscillatory) patterns of breathing, characterized by upper thoracic excursions interspersed with deep (and often irregularly occurring) inspirations. Chronic hyperventilators may trigger a new attack by a single inspiration (Lum, 1976). About two thirds of all chronic hyperventilators have persistently low $PaCO_2$ levels to which the respiratory center has adapted. They are, however, no longer alkalotic.

Changes in inspiratory depth occur with sighing, gasping, exercise, excitement, and fear. Grief-stricken patients sigh; pain can produce a gasp. And each of these changes in rhythmic respirations may set off the symptoms and complex metabolic changes of the syndrome (Magarian, 1982) (Table 1.1).

Acute attacks of hyperventilation may produce cardiovascular changes. In association with a reduced $PaCO_2$ and alkalosis an initial arterial vasodilation occurs, mean BP falls, and both cardiac output and heart rate increase. A few minutes later arterial vasoconstriction (including the coronary arteries) occurs (Kontos, Richardson, Raper, Zubair-Ulhassen, & Patterson, 1972), and the changes in BP, cardiac output, and heart rate disappear.

Hyperventilating patients may manifest sinus tachycardia and arrhythmias at rest, ST-segment elevations or depressions (Tzivoni, Stein, Keren, & Stern, 1980), and supraventricular and ventricular premature beats. Hypocapnic alkalosis reduces coronary arterial blood flow (Neill & Hattenhauer, 1975), and produces coronary vasospasm in patients with and without Prinzmetal's variant angina (Mortensen, Vilhelmson, & Sandoe, 1981), and coronary atherosclerosis. In fact, hyperventilation in some patients may eventuate in MI, probably by producing coronary vasospasm and silent ischemia.

These observations may explain why patients with anxiety and panic disorders have a shortened lifespan (Coryell, Noyes, & Clarcy, 1982; Coryell, Noyes, & House, 1986). At least 50% of all patients diagnosed as having these disorders actually hyperventilate. Thus it seems likely that this functional syndrome—one of ill health—can eventuate in ischemic heart disease and its mortal sequelae (Haines, Imeson, & Meade, 1987).

2) *Functional bowel disorders*. It is of some historical interest that the same physician, DaCosta, who described "soldier's heart" (i.e., the hyperventilation syndrome) also described membranous enteritis, i.e., the functional (irritable) bowel disorder (FBD) in 1871. Be that as it may, this topic is still fraught with confusion and the syndrome goes by a multitude of descriptive names. It has only recently been realized, however,

## TABLE 1.1 Signs and Symptoms of Hyperventilation Syndrome

| | |
|---|---|
| General | Chronic and easy fatigability, weakness, sleep disturbances, headache, excessive sweating, sensation of feeling cold, poor concentration and performance of tasks |
| Neurologic | Numbness and tingling, especially of distal extremities, giddiness, syncope, blurring or tunneling of vision, and impaired thinking |
| Respiratory | Sensation of breathlessness, or inability to take a deep enough breath, with sighing, yawning, and excessive use of upper chest and accessory muscles of respiration, nocturnal dyspnea superficially mimicking paroxysmal nocturnal dyspnea of cardiovascular origin, and nonproductive cough with frequent clearing of throat |
| Cardiovascular | Chest pains, often mimicking angina, palpitations, and tachycardia |
| Gastrointestinal | Aerophagia, resulting in full/bloated sensation, belching, flatus, esophageal reflux and heartburn, sharp lower chest pain, dry mouth, and sensation of lump in throat |
| Musculoskeletal | Myalgias, increased muscle tone with muscle tightness (stiffness), cramps, with occasional carpopedal spasms, and rarely a more generalized tetany |
| Psychiatric | Anxiety, irritability, and tension, though may superficially appear calm (suppression of emotional release), depersonalization, or a feeling of being far away, phobias, and panic attacks |
| Metabolic | Hypocapnia ($PaCO_2$), Alkalosis (in acute, not chronic HVS), Left shift of $O_2$ dissociation curve, Hypophosphatemia (due to intracellular shift), Deionization of $Ca^{2+}$ |
| Renal | Increased excretion of $HCO_3^-$, Increased formation and excretion of ammonium ion and titratable acid, increase in $Na^+$ and $K^+$ |
| Neural | Resetting of respiratory center to low $PaCO_2$, Beta-adrenergic discharge, ? release of histamine |
| Cardiac | Vasodilation followed by constriction, i.e., first fall in mean bp, peripheral resistance, increase in HR & CO, then return to baseline, St-segment depression or elevation, coronary vasoconstriction, sinus arrhythmia or tachycardia, PVCs |
| Cerebrovascular | Vasoconstriction, decreased flow, EEG—High voltage delta activity |

From "Hyperventilation syndrome—In frequently recognized, common expressions of anxiety and stress," by G. J. Magarian, 1982, *Medicine, 61*, p. 224. Copyright 1982 by Williams & Wilkens.

that the putative local variants of FBD ("mucous" or "spastic" colitis) are only a part of a more general functional disturbance of the entire gut with symptoms (Dotevall, Svedlund, & Sjodin, 1982; Lennard-Jones, 1983). What is more, the prevalence of other associated symptoms—headache, backache, muscular aches, chest pain, hyperventilation, anxiety, and depression (in 78%)—do not point to the gut as the sole source of origin of the FBD. The entire distressed person is afflicted. It is also a common disorder: its lifetime prevalence in a population may be 50–75% (Texter & Butler, 1975).

Among the more distressing forms of FBD is gastroesophageal reflux (GER) which may eventuate in esophagitis and esophageal strictures. In GER, gastric acid is cleared less often or forcefully from the esophagus by reflex peristaltic waves. At the same time the lower esophageal sphincter tone is reduced. Because refluxing occurs most frequently at night, sleep recordings have demonstrated that patients with GER awaken too transiently, and do not clear their esophagus or constrict the sphincter. It is thus basically a sleep disorder (Dent et al., 1980).

Related to GER is diffuse esophageal spasm that may be expressed as chest pain and is, therefore, often mistaken for ischemic heart disease. In this form of FBD, nonperistaltic tetanic waves occur in the esophagus and the lower sphincter does not open. A bifurcation (phase transition) in the usual, rhythmic, sequential patterns of esophageal contractions on swallowing has occurred. In other forms of spasm, spontaneous or interrupted contractile rhythms occur. The esophagus can be thrown into tetanic spasm experimentally by stresses (Schuster, 1983). Patients with this disorder are also frequently and diagnosably depressed, anxious, or alcohol abusers.

Rhythmic disturbances occur in the stomach in FBD. The usual rhythmic 3–4 cycle per minute gastric pacemaker potential may be irregular, tetanic, or intermittent at either increased or decreased frequencies (You, Lee, Chey, & Menguy, 1980; You Chey, Lee, Menguy, & Bortoff, 1981). In other patients, jejunal motility and migratory motor complexes (MMC) are irregular or absent. In fact, the MMC is extraordinarily sensitive to any environmental change, including noise and cold. (Motility disturbances occur in animals when stressed: They consist of an inhibition of small bowel contractions and reduced colonic transit time [Williams, Villar, Peterson, & Burks, 1988] which may be due to the release of CRF by the stressor).

The predominantly colonic form of FBD is associated with psychological distress in 80% of all patients. The sources of distress are marital discord, work, and concern about children in persons who are chronic worriers or are always fearful souls (Chaudhary & Truelove, 1962). The distress they experience often takes the form of a depressed mood or a somatization disorder and is present in at least 80% of such patients (Alpers, 1983; Hislop, 1971).

Some of these patients are also unusually sensitive to the pain of abdominal distension (Whitehead, Engel, & Schuster, 1980). They also respond to distension or to the eating of a meal, not by a single contraction, but by tetanic oscillations of the colon (Connell, Jones, & Rowlands, 1965). The electrical activity in the colonic form of FBD in some patients is marked by an increase in the proportion of slow myoelectric activity (Snape & Cohen, 1979). These slow potentials also persist much longer after a meal.

Our knowledge of the psychophysiology of the FBD is far from complete. It is clearly not only a physiological disorder of the gut, but of the whole distressed person. The sources of his/her distress are not fully worked out. And it is obviously not one disorder, because different disturbances of colonic function have been recorded (Weiner, 1988).

## CONCLUSION

An attempt has been made in this chapter to redefine stress, according to Charles Darwin's ideas, and guided by the principles of evolutionary and organismic biology. In so doing, it becomes apparent that stresses are selective pressures with which all creatures have to contend. Not surprisingly, some of these pressures occur because of the fact that animals are social beings—competition and predation are part of the warp and woof of life. Man adds to these selective pressures that are in part occasioned by conflict with his fellow men. Animals are alerted to danger by internal signals, and respond to victory, defeat, and discovery. These responses to selective pressures must be specific and discriminated in order to succeed. The entire organism participates in them. But injury, defeat, infection, and malnutrition may be followed by disease.

Because the organism is one and indivisible, any partial definition of stress "responses" must necessarily fail. Therefore, they cannot be defined only by the physiological response, or by an outdated concept such as disturbed homeostasis. Every function of the organism is oscillatory; no functional (homeostatic) steady-state exists. New concepts are needed to understand how stresses and oscillatory modes of functioning interact.

Because stresses are selective pressures which challenge or threaten whole organisms, one can only study them in intact creatures. Such a line of approach is not traditional in medicine because of its historical concern with material alterations in organs and cells and with the proximate mechanisms of disease. Therefore, a medicine of whole organisms arose, poorly named psychosomatic medicine. The aim of this newer conceptual approach was to study the factors that aided persons in, or prevented them from, meeting or overcoming selective pressures. When they were incapable of doing so, with or without the help of others, profound changes in behavior and physiology occurred. The failure to overcome stresses is experienced by persons as defeat or inability to control the situation and to regulate their behavior and physiology. But the specific mediators of this state of being and the development of disease remain unknown. Thus the pathogenetic puzzle about disease production remains with us. Persons are also "programmed" to develop specific diseases; each program, to add to the complexity of this issue, is not uniform. Thus a comprehensive understanding of the role of stress in disease remains unfulfilled.

However, most persons seen by physicians do not have diseases but are in ill health. The links between stress and the various syndromes of ill health are more tightly forged. These syndromes are characterized by bifurcations (phase transitions) in the usual oscillatory operating modes of basic and vital biological functions.

# REFERENCES

Abraham, R. (1983). Dynamical models for physiology. *American Journal of Physiology, 245*, R467–R472.

Ackerman, S. H. (1981). Premature weaning, thermoregulation and the occurrence of gastric pathology. In H. Weiner, M. A. Hofer, & A. J. Stunkard (Eds.), *Brain, behavior and bodily disease* (pp. 67–86). New York: Raven Press.

Ackerman, S. H. (1987). [Restraint alone can produce gastric erosion formation.] Unpublished observations.

Ackerman, S. H. (1989). Disease consequences of early maternal separation. In H. Weiner, D. Hellhammer, I. Florin, & R. C. Murison (Eds.), *Neuronal control of bodily function: Basic and clinical aspects: Vol. 4: Frontiers of Stress Research* (pp. 85–93). Toronto: Hans Huber.

Ackerman, S. H., Hofer, M. A., & Weiner, H. (1978). Early maternal separation increases gastric ulcer risk in rats by producing latent thermoregulatory disturbance. *Science, 201*, 373–376.

Aloe, L., Alleva, E., Bohm, A., & Levi-Montalcini, R. (1986). Aggressive behavior induces release of nerve growth factor from mouse salivary gland into the bloodstream. *Neurobiology, 83*, 6184–6187.

Alpers, D. H. (1983). Functional gastrointestinal disorders. *Hospital Practice, 18*, 139–153.

Altman, J. (1987). Cerebral cortex: A quiet revolution in thinking. *Nature* (London), *328*, 572–573.

Aravich, P. F., Davis, B. J., Sladek, C. D., Felten, S. Y., & Felten, D. L. (1987). Innervation of the gut: Implications for interaction between the nervous and immune systems. In D. Hellhammer, I. Florin, & H. Weiner (Eds.), *Neuronal control of bodily function: Basic and clinical aspects: Vol. 2: Neurobiological approaches to human disease* (pp. 63–85). Toronto: Hans Huber.

Arthur, R. J. (1982). Life stress and disease: An appraisal of the concept. In L. J. West & M. Stein (Eds.), *Critical issues in behavioral medicine* (pp. 3–17). Philadelphia: J. B. Lippincott.

Ballieux, R. E., & Heijnen, C. J. (1987). Stress and the immune system. In D. Hellhammer, I. Florin & H. Weiner (Eds.), *Neuronal control of bodily function: Basic and clinical aspects: Vol. 2: Neurobiological approaches to human disease* (pp. 301–306). Toronto: Hans Huber.

Beale, N., & Nethercott, S. (1986). Job-loss and health: The influence of age and previous morbidity. *Journal of the Royal College of General Practitioners, 36*, 261–264.

Bernard, C. (1865). *An introduction to the study of experimental medicine*. Translated by H. C. Green, 1957. New York: Dover Publications.

Bernton, E. W., Meltzer, M. S., & Holaday, J. W. (1987). Permissive effects of prolactin on cellular immunity in vivo: Implications relating behavioral stress and host defenses. In D. Hellhammer, I. Florin, & H. Weiner (Eds.), *Neuronal control of bodily function: Basic and clinical aspects: Vol. 2: Neurobiological approaches to human disease* (pp. 290–300). Toronto: Hans Huber.

Bouloux, P. M. G.,& Grossman, A. (1989). Opioid involvement in the neuroendocrine response to stress in humans. In H. Weiner, D. Hellhammer, I. Florin, & R. C. Murison, (Eds.), *Neuronal control of bodily function: Basic and clinical aspects (Vol. 4): Frontiers of stress research* (pp. 209–222). Toronto: Hans Huber.

Brown, M. R., & Fisher, L. (1989). Corticorophin-releasing factor: Regulation of the autonomic nervous system response to stress. In H. Wiener, D. Hellhammer, I. Florin, & R. C. Murison (Eds.), *Neuronal control of bodily function: Basic and clinical aspects: Vol. 4: Frontiers of stress research* (pp. 233–239). Toronto: Hans Huber.

Cannon, W. B. (1929). *Bodily changes in pain, hunger, fear and rage* (2nd ed.). New York: D. Appleton.

Chaudhary, N. A., & Truelove, S. C. (1962). The irritable colon syndrome:

A study of the clinical features, predisposing causes and prognosis in 130 cases. *Quarterly Journal of Medicine, 31*, 307–323.

Connell, A. M., Jones, F. A., & Rowlands, E. N. (1965). Motility of the pelvic colon. IV: Abdominal pain associated with colonic hypermotility after meals. *Gut, 6*, 105–112.

Coryell, W., Noyes, R., & Clarcy, J. (1982). Excess mortality in panic disorder: A comparison with primary unipolar depression. *Archives of General Psychiatry, 39*, 701–703.

Coryell, W., Noyes, R., & House, J. D. (1986). Mortality among outpatients with anxiety disorders. *American Journal of Psychiatry, 143*, 508–510.

Crews, D., & Moore, M. D. (1986). Evolution of mechanisms controlling mating behavior. *Science, 231*, 121–125.

Curtis, G. C., & Nesse, R. (1978). Anxiety and plasma cortisol at the crest of the circadian cycle: Reappraisal of a classical hypothesis. *Psychosomatic Medicine, 40*, 368–378.

Darwin, C. R. (1872). *The expression of the emotions in man and animals*. Reprinted 1965. Chicago: University of Chicago Press.

Dent, J., Dodds, W. J., Friedman, R. H., Sekiguchi, T., Hogan, W. J., Arndorfer, R. C., & Petrie, D. J. (1980). Mechanism of gastroesophageal reflux in recumbent asymptomatic human subjects. *Journal of Clinical Investigation, 65*, 226–267.

Doba, N., & Reis, D. J. (1974). Role of the cerebellum and the vestibular apparatus in regulation of orthostatic reflexes in the cat. *Circulation Research, 34*, 9–14.

Dotevall, G. J., Svedlund, J., & Sjodin, I. (1982). Symptoms in irritable bowel disease. *Scandinavian Journal of Gastroenterology, 17* (Suppl. 79): 16–19.

Drugan, R., Deutsch, S. I., Weizman, A., Weizman, R., Vocci, F. J., Crawley, J. N., Skolnick, P., & Paul, S. M. (1989). Molecular mechanisms of stress and anxiety: Alterations in the benzodiazepine/GABA receptor complex. In H. Weiner, D. Hellhammer, I. Florin, & R. C. Murison (Eds.), *Neuronal control of bodily function: Basic and clinical aspects: Vol. 4: Frontiers of stress research* (pp. 148–159). Toronto: Hans Huber.

Farrow, S. C. (1984). Unemployment and health: A review of methodology. In J. Cullen & J. Siegrist (Eds.), *Breakdown in human adaptation to stress* (pp. 149–158). Boston: Martinus Nijhoff.

Feldman, S. (1989). Afferent neural pathways and hypothalamic neurotransmitters regulating adrenal cortical secretion. In H. Weiner, D. Hellhammer, I. Florin, & R. C. Murison (Eds.), *Neuronal control of bodily function: Basic and clinical aspects: Vol. 4: Frontiers of stress research* (pp. 201–208). Toronto: Hans Huber.

Garfinkel, A. (1983). A mathematics for physiology. *American Journal of Physiology, 245*, R455–R466.

Garrick, T., Veiseh, A., Weiner, H., & Taché, Y. (1988). CRF acts centrally to suppress stimulated gastric contractility in the rat. *Regulatory Peptides*, *21*, 173–181.

Gibbs, D. M. (1986). Vasopressin and oxytocin: Hypothalamic modulators of the stress response. *Psychoneuroendocrinology*, *11*, 131–140.

Gormley, G. J., Lowy, M. T., Reder, A. T., Hospelhorn, V. D., Antel, J. A., & Meltzer, H. Y. (1985). Glucocorticoid receptors in depression: Relationship to the dexamethasone suppression test and mitogen-induced lymphocyte proliferation. *American Journal of Psychiatry*, *142*, 1278–1284.

Grijalva, C., & Roland, B. (1989). The involvement of the hypothalamus and limbic system in the production of stomach erosions. In H. Weiner, D. Hellhammer, I. Florin, & R. C. Murison (Eds.), *Neuronal control of bodily function: Basic and clinical aspects: Vol. 4: Frontiers of stress research* (pp. 72–82). Toronto: Hans Huber.

Grossman, C. J. (1989). Stress and the immune system: Interaction of peptides, gonadal steroids and immune system. In H. Weiner, D. Hellhammer, I. Florin, & R. C. Murison (Eds.), *Neuronal control of bodily function: Basic and clinical aspects: Vol. 4: Frontiers of stress research* (pp. 181–190). Toronto: Hans Huber.

Haines, A. P., Imeson, J. D., & Meade, T. W. (1987). Phobic anxiety and ischemic heart disease. *British Medical Journal*, *295*, 297–299.

Hench, P. S., Kendall, E. C., Slocumb, C. N., & Polley, H. F. (1949). The effect of a hormone of the adrenal cortex (17-hydroxy-11-dehydrocorticosterone: Compound E) and of pituitary adrenocorticotropic hormone on rheumatoid arthritis. *Proceedings of the Staff Meetings of the Mayo Clinic*, *24*, 181–197.

Henry, J. P., & Stephens, P. M. (1977). *Stress, health, and the social environment. A sociobiologic approach to medicine*. New York: Springer Verlag.

Henry, J. P., Stephens, P. M., & Ely, D. (1986). Psychosocial hypertension and the defense and defeat reactions. *Journal of Hypertension*, *4*, 687–697.

Hess, W. R. (1881, 1957). *The functional organization of the diencephalon*. Translated and edited by J. R. Hughes. New York: Grune & Stratton.

Hinkle, L. E., Jr. (1987). Stress and disease: The concept after 50 years. *Social Science and Medicine*, *25*, 561–566.

Hislop, I. G. (1971). Psychological significance of the irritable colon syndrome. *Gut*, *12*, 452–457.

Holaday, J. W. (1989). Opioid peptides: Physiological and behavioral effects. In H. Weiner, D. Hellhammer, I. Florin, & R. C. Murison (Eds.), *Neuronal control of bodily function: Basic and clinical aspects: Vol. 4: Frontiers of stress research* (pp. 309–320). Toronto: Hans Huber.

Irwin, M. R., Vale, W., & Britton, K. (1987). Central corticotropin releasing factor suppresses natural killer cell activity. *Brain, Behavior and Immunity*, *1*, 81–87.

Irwin, M. R., & Weiner, H. (1987). Depressive symptoms and immune functions during bereavement. In S. Zisook (Ed.), *Biopsychosocial aspects of bereavement* (pp. 157–74). Washington, DC: American Psychiatric Press.

Isenberg, J. I., Selling, J. A., Hogan, D. L., & Koss, M. A. (1987). Impaired proximal duodenal mucosal bicarbonate secretion in patients with duodenal ulcer. *New England Journal of Medicine, 316,* 374–379.

Jacobs, S. C. (1987). Psychoendocrine aspects of bereavement. In S. Zisook, (Ed.), *Biopsychosocial aspects of bereavement* (pp. 139–155). Washington, DC: American Psychiatric Press.

Kasl, S. V., Cobb, S., & Brooks, G. W. (1968). Changes in serum uric acid and cholesterol levels in men undergoing job loss. *Journal of the American Medical Association, 206,* 1500–1503.

Kelly, D. D., & Silverman, A.-J. (1988, September). *Plasticity of peptidergic neurons with stress.* Paper presented at The Fourth Annual Symposium on Neuronal Control of Bodily Function: Basic and clinical aspects. Trier, F. R. Germany.

Kontos, H. A., Richardson, D. W., Raper, A. J., Hassen, Z. U., & Patterson, J. L. (1972). Mechanisms of action of hypocapnic alkalosis on limb blood vessels in man and dog. *American Journal of Physiology, 223,* 1296–1307.

Kopin, I. (1989). Adrenergic responses following recognition of stress. In O. Zinder & S. Bresnitz (Eds.), *UCLA Symposia on molecular and cellular biology: Vol. 97. Molecular biology of stress* (pp. 123–132). New York: Alan R. Liss.

LeDoux, J. E. (1989). Central pathways of emotional plasticity. In H. Weiner, D. Hellhammer, I. Florin, & R. C. Murison (Eds.), *Neuronal control of bodily function: Basic and clinical aspects: Vol. 4: Frontiers of stress research* (pp. 122–136). Toronto: Hans Huber.

Lennard-Jones, J. E. (1983). Functional gastrointestinal disorders. *New England Journal of Medicine, 308,* 431–435.

Levi-Montalcini, R. (1987). The nerve growth factor 35 years later. *Science, 237,* 1154–1162.

Levins, R., & Lewontin, R. (1985). *The dialectical biologist.* Cambridge: Harvard University Press.

Lewis, J. W., Cannon, J. T., & Liebeskind, J. C. (1980). Opioid and nonopioid mechanisms of stress-analgesia. *Science, 208,* 623–625.

Lotz, M., Carson, D. A., & Vaughan, J. H. (1987). Substance P activation of rheumatoid synoviocytes: Neural pathway in pathogenesis of arthritis. *Science, 235,* 893–895.

Lum, L. C. (1976). The syndrome of chronic habitual hyperventilation. In O. W. Hill (Ed.), *Modern trends in psychosomatic medicine* (pp. 196–230). London: Butterworth.

Magarian, G. J. (1982). Hyperventilation syndromes: Infrequently recognized common expressions of anxiety and stress. *Medicine, 61,* 219–236.

Mantyh, C. R., Gates, T., Zimmerman, R. P., Kruger, L., Maggio, J. E., Vigna, S. R., Basbaum, A. I., Levine, J., & Mantyh, P. W. (1989). Alterations in density of receptor binding sites for sensory neuropeptides in the spinal cord of arthritic rats. In J. M. Besson & G. R. Guilbaud (Eds.), *The arthritic rat as a model of pain?* (pp. 139–152). Amsterdam: Elsevier.

Meister, B., & Hökfelt, T. (1989). Interaction of peptides and classical neurotransmitters: Focus on neuroendocrine multi-messenger systems. In H. Weiner, D. Hellhammer, I. Florin, & R. C. Murison (Eds.), *Neuronal control of bodily function: Basic and clinical aspects: Vol. 4: Frontiers of stress research* (pp. 160–180). Toronto: Hans Huber.

Morley, J. E. (1989). Neuropeptide-Y: A new stress hormone? In H. Weiner, D. Hellhammer, I. Florin, & R. C. Murison (Eds.), *Neuronal control of bodily function: Basic and clinical aspects: Vol. 4: Frontiers of stress research* (pp. 286–301). Toronto: Hans Huber.

Mortensen, S. A., Vilhelmson, R., & Sandoe, E. (1981). Prinzmetal's variant angina (PVA): Circadian variation in response to hyperventilation. *Acta Medica Scandinavica Suppl. 644*, 38–41.

Munck, A., Guyre, P. M., & Holbrook, N. (1984). Physiological functions of glucocorticoids in stress and their relation to pharmacological actions. *Endocrine Reviews, 5*, 25–44.

Neill, W. A., & Hattenhauer, M. (1975). Impairment of myocardial supply due to hyperventilation. *Circulation, 52*, 854–858.

Norman, G. R., McFarlane, A. H,. & Streiner, D. L. (1985). Patterns of illness among individuals reporting high and low stress. *Canadian Journal of Psychiatry, 30*, 400–405.

Parati, G., Casadei, R., & Mancia, G. (1989). Cardiovascular effects of emotional behavior in animals and humans. In H. Weiner, D. Hellhammer, I. Florin, & R. C. Murison (Eds.), *Neuronal control of bodily function: Basic and clinical aspects: Vol. 4: Frontiers of stress research* (pp. 100–111). Toronto: Hans Huber.

Porreca, F., Sheldon, R. J., & Burks, T. F. (1989). Central and peripheral visceral actions of bombesin. In H. Weiner, D. Hellhammer, I. Florin, & R. C. Murison (Eds.), *Neuronal control of bodily function: Basic and clinical aspects: Vol. 4: Frontiers of stress research* (pp. 276–285). Toronto: Hans Huber.

Rapp, P. E., Mees, A. I. & Sparrow, C. T. (1981). Frequency encoded biochemical regulation is more accurate than amplitude dependent control. *Journal of Theoretical Biology, 90*, 531–544.

Reisine, D. T. (1989). Molecular mechanisms controlling ACTH release. In H. Weiner, D. Hellhammer, I. Florin, & R. C. Murison (Eds.), *Neuronal control of bodily functions: Basic and clinical aspects: Vol. 4: Frontiers of stress research* (pp. 240–249). Toronto: Hans Huber.

Rivier, C. (1989). Effect of the age of the rat and the duration of the stimulus on stress-induced ACTH secretion. In H. Weiner, D. Hellhammer, I. Florin, & R. C. Murison (Eds.), *Neuronal control of bodily function: Basic and clinical aspects: Vol. 4: Frontiers of stress research* (pp. 223–232). Toronto: Hans Huber.

Rivier, C., Rivier, R., & Vale, W. (1986). Stress-induced inhibition of reproductive functions: Role of endogenous corticotropin-releasing factor. *Science, 231*, 607–609.

Saper, C. B. (1989). Role of atrial natriuretic peptide (atriopeptin) in cardiovascular response to stress. In H. Weiner, D. Hellhammer, I. Florin, & R. C. Murison (Eds.), *Neuronal control of bodily function: Basic and clinical aspects: Vol. 4: Frontiers of stress research* (pp. 191–198). Toronto: Hans Huber.

Sapolsky, R. M. (1988). Lessons of the Serengenti: Why some of us are more susceptible to stress. *The Sciences, 28*(3), 38–42.

Sawchenko, P. E. (1989). The functional neuroanatomy of stress related circuitry in the rat brain. In H. Weiner, D. Hellhammer, I. Florin, & R. C. Murison (Eds.), *Neuronal control of bodily function: Basic and clinical aspects: Vol. 4: Frontiers of stress research* (pp. 139–147). Toronto: Hans Huber.

Saxena, K. (1980, February). *Physiological effects of job loss.* Paper presented at the Annual Meeting of the International Society for the Prevention of Stress, Ann Arbor.

Schanberg, S., Evoniuk, G., & Kuhn, C. (1984). Tactile and nutritional aspects of maternal care: Specific regulators of neuroendocrine function and cellular development. *Proceedings of the Society for Experimental Biology and Medicine, 175*, 135–146.

Schleifer, S. J., Keller, S. E., Camarino, M., Thornton, J. C., & Stein, M. (1983). Suppression of lymphocyte stimulation following bereavement. *Journal of the American Medical Association, 250*, 374–377.

Schneiderman, N. (1983). Behavior, autonomic function and animal models of cardiovascular pathology. In T.M. Dembroski & T. H. Schmidt (Eds.), *Biobehavioral bases of coronary heart disease* (pp. 304–364). New York: Karger.

Schuster, M. M. (1983). Disorders of the esophagus: Application of psychophysiological methods to treatment. In R. Holzl & W. E. Whitehead (Eds.). *Psychophysiology of the gastrointestinal tract* (pp. 33–42). New York: Plenum Press.

Selye, H. (1936). A syndrome produced by diverse nocuous agents. *Nature* (London), *148*, 84–85.

Selye, H. (1970). The evolution of the stress concept. *American Scientist, 61*, 692–699.

Shavit, Y., Lewis, J. W., Truman, G. W., Gale, R. P., & Liebeskind, J. D. (1984). Opioid peptides mediate the suppressive effect of stress on natural killer cell cytotoxicity. *Science, 223*, 188–190.

Siegrist, J., Matschinger, H., & Siegrist, K. (1989). Socioemotional inputs to central neuronal regulation of the cardiovascular system. In H. Weiner, D. Hellhammer, I. Florin, & R. C. Murison (Eds.), *Neuronal control of bodily function: Basic and clinical aspects: Vol. 4: Frontiers of stress research* (pp. 174–190). Toronto: Hans Huber.

Smelik, P. G. (1985). Stress and hormones. *Organorama, 22,* 16–18.

Smelik, P. G., Tilders, F. J. H., & Berkenbosch, F. (1989). Participation of adrenaline and vasopressin in the stress response. In H. Weiner, D. Hellhammer, I. Florin, & R. C. Murison (Eds.), *Neuronal control of bodily function: Basic and clinical aspects: Vol. 4: Frontiers of stress research* (pp. 94–99). Toronto: Hans Huber.

Smith, G. R., Jr., Monson, R. A., & Ray, D. C. (1986a). Patients with multiple unexplained symptoms: Their characteristics, functional health and health care utilization. *Archives of Internal Medicine, 146,* 69–72.

Smith, G. R., Jr., Monson, R. A., & Ray, D. C. (1986b). Psychiatric consultation in somatization disorder: A randomized controlled study. *New England Journal of Medicine, 314,* 1407–1413.

Smith, O. A., Astley, C. A., DeVito, J. L., Stein, J. M., & Walsh, K. E. (1980). Functional analysis of hypothalamic control of the cardiovascular responses accompanying emotional behavior. *Federation Proceedings, 39,* 2487–2496.

Smith, W. (1980) Hypothalamic regulation of pituitary secretion of luteinizing hormone: II: Feedback control of gonadotropin secretion. *Bulletin of Mathematical Biology, 42,* 57–78.

Snape, W. J., & Cohen, S. (1979). How colonic motility differs in normal subjects and patients with IBS. *Practical Gastroenterology, 3,* 21–25.

Stephens, R. L., Ishikawa, T., Weiner, H., Novin, D., & Taché, Y. (1988). TRH analogue, RX 77368, microinjected into dorsal vagal complex stimulates gastric secretion in rats. *American Journal of Physiology, 254,* G639–G643.

Stone, E., Bonnet, K., & Hofer, M. A. (1975). Survival and development of maternally deprived rats: Role of body temperature. *Psychosomatic Medicine, 38,* 242–249.

Taché, Y., Goto, Y., LeSiege, D., & Novin, D. (1983). Central nervous system action of thyrotropin-releasing hormone (TRH) to stimulate gastric acid and pepsin secretion in rats. *Endocrinology, 112,* 149.

Taché, Y., Stephens, R. L., & Ishigawa, T. (1989). Stress-induced alterations of gastrointestinal function: Involvement of brain CRF and TRH. In H. Weiner, D. Hellhammer, I. Florin, & R. C. Murison (Eds.), *Neuronal control of bodily functions: Basic and clinical aspects: Vol. 4: Frontiers of stress research* (pp. 265–275). Toronto: Hans Huber.

Texter, E. C., Jr., & Butler, R. C. (1975). The irritable bowel syndrome. *American Family Physician, 11,* 169–173.

Tzivoni, D., Stein, A., Keren, A., & Stern, S. (1980). Electrocardiographic characteristics of neurocirculatory asthenia during everyday activities. *British Heart Journal, 44*, 426–432.

Ursin, H., Baade, E., & Levine, S. (1978). *Psychobiology of stress: A study of coping men.* New York: Academic Press.

Ward, I., & Ward, O. (1989). Reproductive behavior and physiology in prenatally stressed males. In H. Weiner, D. Hellhammer, I. Florin, & R. C. Murison (Eds.), *Neuronal control of bodily function: Basic and clinical aspects: Vol. 4: Frontiers of stress research* (pp. 9–20). Toronto: Hans Huber.

Weiner, H. (1972). Some comments on the transduction of experience by the brain: Implications for our understanding of the relationship of mind to body. *Psychosomatic Medicine, 34*, 355–380.

Weiner, H. (1982). The prospects for psychosomatic medicine: Selected topics. *Psychosomatic Medicine, 44*, 488–517.

Weiner, H. (1985). The concept of stress in the light of studies on disasters, unemployment, and loss: A critical analysis. In M. R. Zales (Ed.), *Stress in health and disease* (pp. 24–94). New York: Brunner/Mazel.

Weiner, H. (1987). Human relationships in health, illness, and disease. In D. Magnusson, and A. Ohman (Eds.), *Psychopathology: An interactional perspective* (pp. 305–323). Orlando, FL: Academic Press.

Weiner, H. (1988). The functional bowel disorders: In H. Weiner & A. Baum (Eds.), *Perspectives in behavioral medicine: Eating regulation and discontrol* (pp. 137–161). Hillsdale, NJ: Lawrence Erlbaum.

Weiner, H., & Mayer, E. (1990). Das Organismus in Gesundheit und Krankheit. (The organism in health and disease). *Psychotherapie Psychosomatik Medizinische Psychologie, 40*, 81–101.

Weiner, H., Thaler, M., Reiser, M. F., & Mirsky, I. A. (1957). Etiology of duodenal ulcer: I: Relation of specific psychological characteristics to rate of gastric secretion. *Psychosomatic Medicine, 19*, 1–10.

Weiss, J. M. (1971). Effects of coping behavior with and without a feedback signal on stress pathology in rats. *Journal of Comparative Physiology and Psychology, 77*, 22–30.

Whitehead, W. E., Engel, B. T., & Schuster, M. M. (1980). Irritable bowel syndrome: Physiological and psychological differences between diarrhea-predominant and constipation-predominant patients. *Digestive Diseases and Sciences, 25*, 404–413.

Williams, C. L., Villar, R. G., Peterson, J. M., & Burks, T. F. (1988). Stress-induced changes in intestinal transit in the rat: A model for irritable bowel syndrome. *Gastroenterology, 94*, 611–621.

Wolff, C. T., Friedman, S. B., Hofer, M. A., & Mason, J. W. (1964). Relationship between psychological defenses and mean urinary 17-hydroxy-corticosteroid excretion rates: I. A predictive study of parents with fatally ill children. *Psychosomatic Medicine, 26*, 576–591.

Yates, F. E. (1982). Outline of a physical theory of physiological systems. *Canadian Journal of Physiology and Pharmacology, 60*, 217–248.

You, C. H., Chey, W. H., Lee, K. T., Menguy, R., & Bortoff, A. (1981). Gastric and small intestinal myoelectric dysrhythmia associated with chronic intractable nausea and vomiting. *Annals of Internal Medicine, 95,* 449–451.

You, C. H., Lee, K. T., Chey, W. H., & Menguy, R. (1980). Electrogastrographic study of patients with unexplained nausea, bloating and vomiting. *Gastroenterology, 79,* 311–314.

Zanchetti, A., Baccelli, G., & Mancia, G. (1976). Fighting, emotion and exercise: Cardiovascular effects in the cat. In G. Onesti, M. Fernandez, and K. E. Kim (Eds.), *Regulation of blood pressure by the central nervous system* (pp. 87–104). New York: Grune & Stratton.

# CHAPTER 2

# Neuroendocrine Aspects of Stress in Major Depression

*Robert T. Rubin*

I T is widely acknowledged that a heterogeneous group of disorders comprises depressive illness; these disorders have differing clinical symptom pictures and they respond to different treatment modalities. Many individuals suffer self-limited depressions, often precipitated by a major life stress. However, there is a particular type of depression, termed endogenous (Kendell, 1976; Spitzer, Endicott, & Robins, 1978) or melancholic (American Psychiatric Association [APA], 1980, 1987), that is characterized by a specific set of symptoms, a protracted course, often a family history of similar illness, and generally a responsiveness to somatic therapies.

The signs and symptoms of endogenous or melancholic depression have been codified in the criterion-based diagnostic systems introduced into psychiatry since the early 1970s (APA, 1980, 1987; Feighner, Robins, Guze, Woodruff, Winokur, & Munoz, 1972; Spitzer et al., 1978), but the diagnostic algorithm, i.e., the specific number and combination of criteria necessary to support the diagnosis, has changed dramatically. This is clearly evident in the difference between "melancholia" according to the DSM-III (APA, 1980), for which pervasive anhedonia and lack of reactivity to pleasurable stimuli must both be present, along with three of six other signs and symptoms, and the "melancholic type" according to the DSM-III-R (APA, 1987), in which any five of nine criteria must be present. These may or not include the two *sine qua non* criteria of DSM-III melancholia listed above.

The reasons for this change include both the availability of newer research data and compromise among members of the committees established to rewrite the DSM (Zimmerman & Spitzer, 1989). Nevertheless, an important fundamental conceptual shift resulting from the establishment of a criterion-based DSM has been the elimination of absence of antecedent stress as a distinguishing feature in the diagnosis of melancholic major depression, in contrast to its importance in the older neurotic vs. endogenous depression dichotomy. It is now recognized that precipitating stresses may or may not be evident in the histories of melancholic depressives and do not themselves determine the nature of the syndrome.

Major depression, especially the endogenous or melancholic subtype as variously defined above, not infrequently has associated neuroendocrine disturbances (Carroll, 1978; Checkley, 1980; Rubin, 1989; Rubin, Gouin, & Poland, 1973; Rubin & Poland, 1982, 1983). These include abnormalities in the secretion patterns of several of the anterior pituitary polypeptide hormones and their peripheral target endocrine gland hormones. The most clearly delineated of these are in the hypothalamo-pituitary-adrenal cortical (HPA) axis—hypersecretion of ACTH and cortisol, and inadequate suppression of cortisol following administration of the synthetic glucocorticoid, dexamethasone. Other reported neuroendocrine abnormalities are reduced nocturnal TSH secretion and a blunted TSH response to TRH administration, reduced growth hormone responses to adrenergic challenges such as clonidine and desipramine administration, and perhaps reduced prolactin responses to opioidergic and serotonergic challenges such as morphine and fenfluramine.

Key questions concerning these neuroendocrine changes relate to their origin; i.e., are they specific to the depressive syndrome, or do they occur in other psychiatric illnesses? (Similar changes can occur, for example, in anorexia nervosa.) Can these changes be traced to any specific neurotransmitter or neuromodulator abnormalities in the central nervous system (CNS)? And, of importance to the emphasis of this chapter, is a common denominator of the neuroendocrine changes a more-or-less nonspecific stress factor? In this selective review, the consideration will be the relationship of stress to HPA axis function in major depression, because this neuroendocrine axis is the most robustly affected in this illness, and for decades it has been a major focus of neuroendocrine stress research.

## LIMBIC–HYPOTHALAMIC–PITUITARY RELATIONSHIPS

The pituitary gland is under the major influence of the brain, through a number of neurotransmitter actions on the synthesis and release of the "hypothalamo-hypophysiotropic hormones." These releasing and inhibiting factors, made in specialized neurosecretory cells in the hypothalamus, are transported to the hypophysis (anterior pituitary) via the pituitary portal circulation and effect the release, or inhibition of release, of the anterior pituitary hormones. Several of these hypothalamic hormones have been characterized and synthesized for use in endocrine challenge tests; they include corticotropin (ACTH)-releasing hormone (CRH), thyrotropin (TSH)-releasing hormone (TRH), growth hormone-releasing hormone (GHRH) and inhibiting hormone (somatostatin), and gonadotropin (luteinizing hormone [LH] and follicle-stimulating hormone [FSH])-releasing hormone (GnRH). These hypothalamic hormones may have more than one action. For example, TRH can promote the secretion of both TSH and prolactin, and somatostatin can inhibit the secretion of both growth hormone and TSH.

Neural inputs to the hypothalamus come from many areas of the brain, especially the limbic system. The neurotransmitter regulation of the pituitary hormone releasing and inhibiting factors is extremely complex (Tuomisto & Männistö, 1985). Some neurotransmitters appear to be involved in a primary way; for example, dopamine itself most likely is prolactin-inhibiting factor. More than one neurotransmitter can affect the neurons producing a given hypothalamic hormone; for example, norepinephrine (NE) inputs appear to be inhibitory, and serotonin inputs to be stimulatory, to CRH secretion. The effects of these neurotransmitters on the other releasing and inhibiting factors can be quite varied. And other neurotransmitters and neuromodulators may be secondarily involved, for example, opioid modulation of the influence of the various biogenic amines on hypothalamic hormone secretion. Finally, other hormones may interact with the releasing and inhibiting factors in their effects on pituitary hormone secretion; for example, the posterior pituitary hormone, vasopressin, can synergize with CRH to stimulate ACTH production.

## CONCEPTS OF PSYCHOENDOCRINE RESPONSES TO STRESS

Some 50 years ago, Hans Selye proposed the concept of the general adaptation syndrome, based on his finding of a consistent HPA axis activation in response to many kinds of physical and psychological stimuli (Selye, 1973). The first component was a triad of physiologic responses, described by Selye as the "alarm reaction," which included enlargement and hyperemia of the adrenals with loss of their corticosteroid-laden lipid content, marked atrophy of the thymus and lymph glands, and ulceration of the gastric mucosa. We now know that the latter two phenomena (involution of lymphoid tissue and stress ulcers) can be sequelae of increased circulating glucocorticoids, as well as of a direct influence of the autonomic nervous system.

In a series of studies in monkeys adapted to restraining chairs, Mason and coworkers (Mason, 1968a, 1971, 1975) measured a panoply of hormone responses to noxious stimuli, including the stress of being placed in the chair for the first time. While the findings of these studies, conducted over about two decades, were numerous, two overarching concepts resulted from the data in aggregate. The first was that the various endocrine axes responded to the various stresses in a coordinated way, with some hormone concentrations in blood increasing rapidly during the time of the stress and decreasing thereafter, while other hormones either did not increase, or were even suppressed, during the stress. Those hormones which showed a rapid increase were the so-called "catabolic" hormones—glucocorticoids, epinephrine, norepinephrine, growth hormone—which help mobilize stored energy in order to support the body's physiologic response to the stress (in natural situations, the "fight or flight" response) (Cannon, 1963). Those hormones whose secretion, in contrast, was not increased until after the stress had ended and levels of the first group of hormones had begun to decrease, were the "anabolic" hormones—insulin, estrogens, testosterone, androgenic metabolites—which help rebuild body tissues that had been broken down during the earlier, immediate need for energy. Thus, psychoendocrine responses to stress are temporally organized in a way which allows greatest synergism among the various hormones and counters their potentially antagonistic physiological effects. Mason and coworkers thus expanded the work of Cannon on the adrenal medullary hormones, epinephrine and norepinephrine, and the work of Selye on the adrenal cortex, by including the stress responses of other hormones that could be measured reliably at the time.

Additionally, these investigators further studied the putative nonspecificity of the stress response by exposing monkeys to both physical and psychological stresses, the two exposures being separate as they could be in the laboratory. From this work the second overarching concept emerged, which was that different stresses, physical and psychological, do not produce the same hormone secretion patterns; i.e., there is specificity to the psychoendocrine response (Mason, 1968a, 1971). For example, a sudden increase in heat in the laboratory produced an increase in adrenal cortical hormone production, whereas a slow increase to the same temperature, which did not pose a perceptible threat, resulted in a decrease in adrenal cortical activity, consonant with the changed metabolic demands upon the animal. Similarly, fasting of monkeys in a laboratory in which the monkeys could see and hear other animals being fed produced an adrenal cortical stress response, whereas giving these monkeys non-nutritive food pellets at the times of regular feeding resulted in no such hormone response. This concept of the specificity of cortisol responses to stress is important in considering the etiology of the HPA axis hyperactivity in depression and its relationship to stress in a nonspecific (nonsyndromally related) way, as will be discussed below.

## PUTATIVE NEUROTRANSMITTER ABNORMALITIES IN MAJOR DEPRESSION

Research on the pathogenesis of depression has begun to emphasize the likelihood that no single neurotransmitter system is disordered in depression; rather, multiple neurotransmitters are likely to be involved, either directly or by indirect effects, in the etiology of depression and in its response to antidepressant drugs (Risby, Hsiao, Sunderland, Ågren, Rudorfer, & Potter, 1987). The notion that depression is due to an excess or deficiency of a single neuroregulator (e.g., the norepinephrine (NE) depletion model of depression) may be of less heuristic value than the concept that neurotransmitter-receptor systems are dysregulated (Siever & Davis, 1985).

### Norepinephrine (NE) Systems

Central NE systems have long been hypothesized to be abnormal in depression. However, the original hypothesis of a central NE deficit state in depression (Bunney & Davis, 1965; Schildkraut, 1965) has not been fully supported. Indeed, the more consistent finding has been that unipolar depressives (those without a history of mania) often have increased CNS and peripheral NE activity relative to controls, as shown by increased plasma and CSF concentrations and urinary excretion of the NE metabolite, 3-methoxy-4-hydroxyphenylglycol (MHPG) (Potter, Rudorfer, & Goodwin, 1987). On the other hand, depressed bipolar patients show reduced NE activity relative to unipolar patients.

NE receptors also appear to differ between depressed patients and controls. Postmortem studies of suicide completers, many of whom were depressed, have revealed a 73% increase in CNS $\beta$-receptor binding (Mann, Stanley, McBride, & McEwen, 1986). Most studies of chronic antidepressant treatment in animals indicate that $\beta$ receptors become down-regulated (Charney, Menkes, & Heninger, 1981). Platelet $\alpha_2$-receptor binding appears to be increased in depression (Doyle, George, Ravindron, & Philpott, 1985; Garcia-Sevilla, Zis, Hollingsworth, Greden, & Smith, 1981). In contrast, central $\alpha_2$ receptors appear to be less sensitive to agonist stimulation, as evidenced by a blunted growth hormone (GH) response and a lack of reduction in plasma MHPG following administration of the $\alpha_2$ agonist clonidine to depressed patients (Charney, Heninger, Sternberg, Hafstad, Giddings, & Landis, 1982; Siever et al., 1982, Siever, Uhde, Jimerson, Post, Lake, & Murphy, 1984). While the data on changes in NE systems are complex and some studies conflict, one current hypothesis of the pathogenesis of depression is that the $\alpha_2$ receptor is subsensitized by persistent elevations in central NE.

## Serotonin Systems

Dysregulation of central serotonergic systems also has been suggested to occur in depression. The major metabolite of serotonin, 5-hydroxyindoleacetic acid (5-HIAA), is often reduced in the CSF of depressives and suicidal patients (Åsberg, Träskman, & Thorén, 1976). Other components of serotonin systems also are altered. Tritiated imipramine binding sites on blood platelets have been found to be reduced during an episode of depression and appear to return to normal with recovery (Briley, Langer, Raisman, Sechter, & Zarifian, 1980; Roy, Everett, Pickar, & Paul, 1987). Serotonin$_2$ receptor binding has been reported to be increased in cortical brain tissue from suicide victims (Stanley & Mann, 1983). These findings are compatible with the hypothesis that serotonin turnover is reduced in depression, along with compensatory changes in pre- and postsynaptic receptors.

## Other Systems

Central cholinergic systems also have been reported to be dysregulated in depressive illness. While data on changes in acetylcholine receptor binding in depressives and suicide victims have been inconsistent, depressives are more sensitive than controls to challenge with cholinergic agonists. Physostigmine challenge has been shown to produce significantly greater secretion of ACTH and cortisol in depressives than in controls (Risch, Janowsky, & Gillin, 1983). Other, possibly relevant, CNS neuroregulators that may be disordered in depression, and perhaps related to the observed neuroendocrine abnormalities in depression, are changes in dopaminergic (Swerdlow & Koob, 1987) and opioidergic systems.

# HYPOTHALAMO-PITUITARY-ADRENAL CORTICAL (HPA) AXIS ABNORMALITIES IN MAJOR DEPRESSION

As mentioned earlier, the most prominent of the abnormalities of neuro-endocrine function in major depression is an overactivity of the HPA axis, as reflected by increased circulating ACTH and cortisol concentrations (Carroll, Curtis, & Mendels, 1976a; Pfohl, Sherman, Schlechte, & Stone, 1985; Rubin, Poland, Lesser, Winston, & Blodgett, 1987), increased cerebrospinal fluid cortisol concentrations (Carroll, Curtis, & Mendels, 1976b; Träskman, Tybring, Åsberg, Bertillson, Lantto, & Schalling, 1980), increased urinary free cortisol excretion (Carroll, 1976; Carroll, Curtis, & Mendels, 1976c; Carroll, Curtis, Davies, Mendels & Sugarman, 1976), and cortisol resistance to dexamethasone suppression (Arana, Baldessarini, & Ornsteen, 1985; Carroll, 1985; Carroll et al., 1981; Holsboer, 1983; Rubin & Poland, 1984). Considerable work has been done attempting to develop a clinical application for these hormone changes as biological state markers of endogenous depression; in this regard, the dexamethasone suppression test (DST) has been the most thoroughly investigated "biological test" in psychiatry to date.

Only a few studies have addressed more fundamental issues of HPA axis regulation in depression, such as the relationship between pre-DST cortisol hypersecretion and DST outcome. Because less-than-perfect relationships between various pre-DST measures of cortisol and DST status have been found, there has been some controversy as to where in the HPA axis the physiologic stimulus to cortisol hypersecretion occurs. For example, we studied HPA axis function in 40 primary definite endogenous depressives and 40 normal matched control subjects (Rubin, Poland, Lesser, Winston, & Blodgett, 1987) and found the following: 15 patients (38%) were DST nonsuppressors. These 15 nonsuppressors had significantly higher pre-DST serum and urine cortisol measures during both the day and the night than both their matched controls and the 25 suppressor patients. All cortisol measures were unimodally distributed across both groups of subjects. Circadian cortisol rhythms of similar magnitude occurred in both groups, and there was no significant phase advance of the circadian rhythm in the patients. And the cortisol measures before and after dexamethasone administration were positively correlated to a similar degree in the patients and the control subjects.

This latter finding suggests that pre-DST HPA hyperactivity and cortisol nonsuppression on the DST are not independently physiologically regulated in endogenous depression, as has been suggested by others on the basis of only partial overlap between increased pre-DST circulating cortisol and a positive DST (Rubin, Poland, Lesser, Winston, & Blodgett, 1987). Further evidence against this hypothesis is provided by the correspondence in depressed patients between ACTH and cortisol concentrations, both before and after dexamethasone (Mortola, Liu, Gillin, Rasmussen, & Yen, 1987; Pfohl, Sherman, Schlechte, & Stone, 1985). The overall results of our study, and of other studies in aggregate, suggest that depressed patients, especially DST nonsuppressors, have a higher cortisol secretion than normal subjects, even occasionally in the Cushingoid range, but they have preservation of the timing and amplitude of their cortisol circadian rhythm, in contrast to many patients with Cushing's syndrome. This may be one reason why depressed patients with cortisol hypersecretion manifest few, if any, physical and laboratory stigmata of Cushing's syndrome.

Challenge studies with CRH also have revealed important information about HPA axis function in depression. Most of the studies have shown a decreased ACTH response to CRF in depressed patients compared to control subjects, indicating some down-regulation of CRH receptors on the corticotrophs of the pituitary (Gold & Chrousos, 1985; Holsboer et al., 1984). This suggests increased endogenous CRH production. The cortisol response following CRH, on the other hand, has been for the most part similar between depressives and controls, even though the depressives had a blunted ACTH response, suggesting the possibility of up-regulation of ACTH receptors in the adrenal cortex. The adrenals of depressed patients and suicide victims have been reported to be larger than those of controls (Dorovini-Zis & Zis, 1987; Nemeroff et al., 1992; Rubin, Phillips, Sadow, & McCracken, 1992). All these data taken together provide consistent evidence for increased limbic-hypothalamic driving of the HPA axis in endogenous depression, resulting in some down-regulation of CRH receptors in the pituitary but increased circulating ACTH concentrations nevertheless. The increased ACTH secretion results in increased circulating cortisol concentrations at all times of the day and night, but, as mentioned, with preservation of the timing and amplitude of the normal cortisol circadian rhythm.

Because the same putative central nervous system (CNS) neurotransmitters appear to be involved in both the modulation of affects and the regulation of the hypothalamic releasing and inhibiting factors, it is tempting to suggest that a common CNS neurotransmitter dysfunction underlies both the depressive state and the altered HPA axis dynamics. However, proposing this hypothesis has been considerably easier than demonstrating it. For example, as mentioned, an NE deficiency hypothesis of depression has been proposed (Bunney & Davis, 1965; Schildkraut, 1965), and NE neurotransmission in the hypothalamus has been considered to be inhibitory to CRH secretion and thus to ACTH and cortisol secretion (VanLoon, 1973; Weiner & Ganong, 1978). It is logical to consider that depressives with hyperactivity of the HPA axis may represent those having a deficiency of NE function in the CNS underlying their affective disorder, and it would further logically follow that such patients should respond to antidepressants which enhance CNS noradrenergic neurotransmission better than they would respond to antidepressants which affect primarily serotonin or other neurotransmitters.

However, in clinical practice this has not proved to be the case; reports which have suggested a differential response to antidepressants in DST-positive and DST-negative patients have been countered by a number of other reports indicating that there is no difference in antidepressant response between DST-positive and DST-negative depressives (cf. Rubin, 1989, for references). One complicating factor is that antidepressants which may have selective effects on particular neurotransmitters in laboratory test situations have much more widespread effects in treated patients. For example, desmethylimipramine (a fairly specific presynaptic NE uptake inhibitor), zimelidine (a specific serotonin uptake inhibitor), and clorgyline (a monoamine oxidase-A inhibitor), when given to patients for several weeks, all reduced both the NE metabolite, MHPG, and the serotonin metabolite, 5-HIAA, in the cerebrospinal fluid (Potter et al., 1985). Because of the intricate functional interrelationships among many neurotransmitter systems in the CNS, there is little wonder that measures of HPA axis hyperactivity thus far have not been able to predict which depressed patient will respond to which antidepressant.

## INFLUENCE OF STRESS ON HPA AXIS ACTIVITY IN MAJOR DEPRESSION

Because of the impetus given to psychoendocrine research by Selye's formulation of the general adaptation syndrome, as discussed above, and because blood and urine corticosteroid measurement techniques were available in the 1950s, early endocrine studies of depression focused on the HPA axis (Mason, 1968b; Rubin & Mandell, 1966). These studies were consistent in their results that HPA activity was increased compared to mania or normalcy. Some investigators believed that the subjectively experienced anxiety and dysphoria of the depressed patient resulted in an adrenal cortical stress response according to the Selye model (Sachar,

1975), while others postulated that both the depressed affect and the increased corticosteroid secretion could be secondary to an underlying disturbance of brain function (Carroll, 1976; Rubin & Mandell, 1966), as considered above. Studies of the circadian pattern of cortisol secretion in endogenous/melancholic depression support the latter hypothesis, that a CNS mechanism more fundamental than subjectively felt anxiety appears to underlie the increased corticosteroid production, because increased HPA axis activity occurs in apathetic as well as in anxious depressives, and it occurs throughout the entire 24 hours, as discussed above.

There has been an undercurrent of concern that certain elements of the management of depressed patients could be considered stressful and thereby might affect HPA axis function. One important consideration is the stress of hospitalization; this has been suggested to contribute to increased HPA axis activity in patients who were studied when newly hospitalized (cf. Rubin, Poland, Lesser, Martin, Blodgett, & Winston, 1987 for references). Any such contribution, however, appears to be mild at best; for example, in our 40 endogenous depressives, about half of whom were inpatients and half outpatients at the time of study, we found no relationship of this variable to the cortisol measures (Rubin, Poland, Lesser, Martin, Blodgett, & Winston, 1987).

There have been several studies in which DST results, as a measure of HPA axis activity, have been related to individual Hamilton depression scale (Hedlund & Vieweg, 1979) item scores, in an attempt to discern which symptom components of the depressive syndrome are most strongly correlated with neuroendocrine changes. The results have been quite disparate, most likely due to the large number of symptom items analyzed versus the numbers of patients included in these studies (cf. Rubin, Poland, Lesser, Martin, Blodgett, & Winston, 1987 for references). In order to reduce the number of independent variables, we used previously developed factor items of the Hamilton depression scale (Rhoades & Overall, 1983) to relate to the HPA axis measures in our 40 depressives; this reduced the number of independent variables from 21 individual items to seven factors. The agitation/anxiety factor showed a modest but consistent positive correlation with the pre-dexamethasone serum and urine cortisol measures, but no such correlation with the DST results. These results suggested that endogenous depressives may indeed have a neurotransmitter disturbance resulting in increased activity of the HPA axis (Rubin & Poland, 1984), but they also appear to have an additional increment of HPA hyperactivity as a result of the subjective experience of anxiety. That is to say, even moderate to severe endogenous depressives can still respond to their illness with a subjective dysphoria that adds an additional stress response component to their fundamental neuroendocrine dysregulation. The final degree of HPA axis activation in depression thus appears to be multidetermined.

## CONCLUSIONS

In conclusion, there is little chance that there will be a simple correspondence found between specific symptom components of the depressive syndrome, such as dimensions of depression or anxiety, and a specific neuroendocrine alteration, such as hyperactivity of the HPA axis. The neurotransmitter regulation of both the affective disturbance and the various neuroendocrine axes is too complex for such a reductionistic search to be fruitful. In future studies we should pursue a multivariate approach, both toward the psychiatric manifestations, by using multiple diagnostic systems (Kendell, 1982) and robust psychopathological dimensions such as those offered by factor analysis of well-characterized rating scales, and toward the neuroendocrine alterations, by evaluating multiple hormone systems (Rubin, Heist, McGeoy, Hanada, & Lesser, 1992; Rubin, Poland, & Lesser, 1989, 1990; Rubin, Poland, Lesser, & Martin, 1987; Rubin, Poland, Lesser, & Martin, 1989; Rubin, Poland, Lesser, Winston, & Blodgett, 1987). Such studies require large sample sizes in order to achieve stable, replicable data. They are tedious and expensive, but there is no alternative for the continued exploration of the neuroendocrinology of affective disorders and the importance of stress in this pathophysiological process.

## ACKNOWLEDGMENT

Supported in part by NIMH Research Scientist Award MH 47363 and by NIMH research grant MH 28380.

## REFERENCES

American Psychiatric Association. (1980). *Diagnostic and statistical manual of mental disorders (3rd ed.)*. Washington, DC.

American Psychiatric Association. (1987). *Diagnostic and statistical manual of mental disorders (3rd ed. rev.)*. Washington, DC.

Amsterdam, J. D. Marinelli, D. L., Arger, P., & Winokur, A. (1987). Assessment of adrenal gland volume by computed tomography in depressed patients and healthy volunteers: A pilot study. *Psychiatry Research, 21*, 189–197.

Arana, G. W., Baldessarini, R. J., & Ornsteen, M. (1985). The dexamethasone suppression test for diagnosis and prognosis in psychiatry: Commentary and review. *Archives of General Psychiatry, 42*, 1193–1204.

Åsberg, M., Träskman, L., & Thorén, P. (1976). 5-HIAA in the cerebrospinal fluid: A biochemical suicide predictor? *Archives of General Psychiatry, 33*, 1193–1204.

Briley, M. S., Langer, S. Z., Raisman, R., Sechter, D., & Zarifian, E. (1980). Tritiated imipramine binding sites are decreased in platelets of untreated depressed patients. *Science, 209*, 303–305.

Bunney, W. E., Jr., & Davis, J. M. (1965). Norepinephrine in depressive reactions: A review. *Archives of General Psychiatry, 13*, 483–494.

Cannon, W. B. (1963). *The Wisdom of the body*. New York: Norton.

Carroll, B. J. (1976). Limbic system-adrenal cortex regulation in depression and schizophrenia. *Psychosomatic Medicine, 38*, 106–121.

Carroll, B. J. (1978). Neuroendocrine function in affective disorders. In M. A. Lipton, A. DiMascio, & K. F. Killam (Eds.), *Psychopharmacology: A generation of progress* (pp. 487–497). New York: Raven Press.

Carroll, B. J. (1985). Dexamethasone suppression test: A review of contemporary confusion. *Journal of Clinical Psychiatry, 46*, 13–24.

Carroll, B. J., Curtis, G. C., & Mendels, J. (1976a). Neuroendocrine regulation in depression: I. Limbic system-adrenocortical dysfunction. *Archives of General Psychiatry, 33*, 1039–1044.

Carroll, B. J., Curtis, G. C., & Mendels, J. (1976b). Cerebrospinal fluid and plasma free cortisol concentrations in depression. *Psychological Medicine, 6*, 235–244.

Carroll, B. J., Curtis, G. C., Davies, B. M., Mendels, J., & Sugerman, A. A. (1976). Urinary free cortisol excretion in depression. *Psychological Medicine, 6*, 43–50.

Carroll, B. J., Curtis, G. C., & Mendels, J. (1976c). Neuroendocrine regulation in depression: II. Discrimination of depressed from non-depressed patients. *Archives of General Psychiatry, 33*, 1051–1058.

Carroll, B. J., Feinberg, M., Greden, J. F., Tarika, J., Albala, A. A., Haskett, R. F., James, N. M., Kronfol, Z., Lohr, N., Steiner, M., de Vigne, J. P., & Young, E. (1981). A specific laboratory test for the diagnosis of melancholia: Standardization, validation, and clinical utility. *Archives of General Psychiatry, 38*, 15–22.

Charney, D. S., Heninger, G. R., Sternberg, D. E., Hafstad, K. M., Giddings, S., & Landis, H. (1982). Adrenergic receptor sensitivity in depression. *Archives of General Psychiatry, 39*, 290–294.

Charney, D. S., Menkes, D. B., & Heninger, G. R. (1981). Receptor sensitivity and the mechanism of action of antidepressant treatment. *Archives of General Psychiatry, 38,* 1160–1180.

Checkley, S. A. (1980). Neuroendocrine tests of monoamine function in man: A review of basic theory and its application to the study of depressive illness. *Psychological Medicine, 10,* 35–53.

Dorovini-Zis, K., & Zis, A. P. (1987). Increased adrenal weight in victims of violent suicide. *American Journal of Psychiatry, 144,* 1214–1215.

Doyle, M. C., George, A. J., Ravindran, A. V., & Philpott, R. (1985). Platelet $\alpha_2$-adrenoreceptor binding in elderly depressed patients. *American Journal of Psychiatry, 142,* 1489–1490.

Feighner, J. P., Robins, E., Guze, S. B., Woodruff, R. A., Jr., Winokur, G., & Munoz, R. (1972). Diagnostic criteria for use in psychiatric research. *Archives of General Psychiatry, 26,* 57–63.

Garcia-Sevilla, J. A., Zis, A. P., Hollingsworth, P. J., Greden, J. F., & Smith, C. B. (1981). Platelet $\alpha_2$-adrenergic receptors in major depressive disorder: Binding of tritiated clonidine before and after tricyclic antidepressant drug treatment. *Archives of General Psychiatry, 38,* 1327–1333.

Gold, P. W., & Chrousos, G. P. (1985). Clinical studies with corticotropin releasing factor: Implications for the diagnosis and pathophysiology of depression, Cushing's disease, and adrenal insufficiency. *Psychoneuroendocrinology, 10,* 401–419.

Hedlund, J. L., & Vieweg, B. W. (1979). The Hamilton rating scale for depression: A comprehensive review. *Journal of Operational Psychiatry, 10,* 149–165.

Holsboer, F. (1983). The dexamethasone suppression test in depressed patients: Clinical and biochemical aspects. *Journal of Steroid Biochemistry, 19,* 251–257.

Holsboer, F., Müller, O. A., Doerr, H. G., Sippell, W. G., Stalla, G. K., Gerken, A., Steiger, A. M., & Boll, E. (1984). ACTH and multisteroid responses to corticotropin-releasing factor in depressive illness: Relationship to multisteroid responses after ACTH stimulation and dexamethasone suppression. *Psychoneuroendocrinology, 9,* 147–160.

Kendell, R. E. (1976). The classification of depressions: A review of contemporary confusion. *British Journal of Psychiatry, 129,* 15–28.

Kendell, R. E. (1982). The choice of diagnostic criteria for biological research. *Archives of General Psychiatry, 39,* 1334–1339.

Mann, J. J., Stanley, M., McBride, A., & McEwen, B. S. (1986). Increased serotonin$_2$ and beta-adrenergic receptor binding in the frontal cortices of suicide victims. *Archives of General Psychiatry, 43,* 954–959.

Mason, J. W. (1968a). Organization of psychoendocrine mechanisms. *Psychosomatic Medicine, 30,* 565–808.

Mason, J. W. (1968b). A review of psychoendocrine research on the pituitary-adrenal cortical system. *Psychosomatic Medicine, 30,* 576–607.

Mason, J. W. (1971). A re-evaluation of the concept of "non-specificity" in stress theory. *Journal of Psychiatric Research, 8*, 323–333.

Mason, J. W. (1975). Emotion as reflected in patterns of endocrine integration. In L. Levi (Ed.), *Emotions: Their parameters and measurement* (pp. 143–181). New York: Raven Press.

Mortola, J. F., Liu, J. H., Gillin, J. C., Rasmussen, D. D., & Yen, S. S. C. (1987). Pulsatile rhythms of adrenocorticotropin (ACTH) and cortisol in women with endogenous depression: Evidence for increased ACTH pulse frequency. *Journal of Clinical Endocrinology and Metabolism, 65*, 962–968.

Nemeroff, C. B., Krishnan, K. R. R., Reed, D., Leder, R., Beam, C., & Dunnick, N. R. (1992). Adrenal gland enlargement in major depression: A computed tomographic study. *Archives of General Psychiatry, 49*, 384–387.

Pfohl, B., Sherman, B., Schlechte, J., & Stone, R. (1985). Pituitary/adrenal axis rhythm disturbances in psychiatric depression. *Archives of General Psychiatry, 42*, 897–903.

Potter, W. Z., Rudorfer, M. V., & Goodwin, F. K. (1987). Biological findings in bipolar disorders. In R. E. Hales & A. J. Frances (Eds.), *The American Psychiatric Association annual review* (pp. 32–60). Washington, DC: APA Press.

Potter, W. Z., Scheinin, M., Golden, R. N., Rudorfer, M. V., Cowdry, R., Calil, H. M., Ross, R. J., Linnoila, M. (1985). Selective antidepressants and cerebrospinal fluid: Lack of specificity on norepinephrine and serotonin metabolites. *Archives of General Psychiatry, 42*, 1171–1177.

Rhoades, H. M., & Overall, J. E. (1983). The Hamilton Depression Scale: Factor scoring and profile classification. *Psychopharmacology Bulletin, 19*, 91–96.

Risby, E. D., Hsiao, J. K., Sunderland, T., Ågren, H., Rudorfer, M. V., & Potter, W. Z. (1987). The effects of antidepressants in the cerebrospinal fluid homovanillic acid/5-hydroxy-indoleacetic acid ratio. *Clinical Pharmacology and Therapeutics, 42*, 547–554.

Risch, S. C., Janowsky, D. S., & Gillin, J. C. (1983). Muscarinic supersensitivity of anterior pituitary ACTH and beta-endorphin release in major depressive illness. *Peptides, 4*, 789–792.

Roy, A., Everett, D., Pickar, D., & Paul, S. M. (1987). Platelet tritiated imipramine binding and serotonin uptake in depressed patients and controls: Relationship to plasma cortisol levels before and after dexamethasone administration. *Archives of General Psychiatry, 44*, 320–327.

Rubin, R. T. (1989). Pharmacoendocrinology of major depression. *European Archives of Psychiatry and Neurological Sciences, 238*, 259–267.

Rubin, R. T., Gouin, P. R., & Poland, R. E. (1973). Biogenic amine metabolism and neuroendocrine function in affective disorders. In R. de la Fuente & M. N. Weisman (Eds.), *Psychiatry: Proceedings of the V World Congress of Psychiatry* (pp. 1036–1039). Princeton, NJ: Excerpta Medica.

Rubin, R. T., Heist, E. K., McGeoy, S. S., Hanada, K., & Lesser, I. M. (1992). Neuroendocrine aspects of primary endogenous depression: XI.

Serum melatonin measures in patients and matched control subjects. *Archives of General Psychiatry, 49*, 558–567.

Rubin, R. T., & Mandell, A. J. (1966). Adrenal cortical activity in pathological emotional states: A review. *American Journal of Psychiatry, 123*, 387–400.

Rubin, R. T., Phillips, J. J., Sadow, T. F., & McCracken, J. T. (1992). Adrenal cortical volume in major depression: Increase during the depressive episode and decrease with successful treatment. Abstract of Thirty-first Annual Meeting of the American College of Neuropsychopharmacology, p. 90.

Rubin, R. T., & Poland, R. E. (1982). The chronoendocrinology of endogenous depression. In E. E. Müller & R. MacLeod (Eds.), *Neuroendocrine perspectives: Vol. 1* (pp. 305–337). Amsterdam: Elsevier.

Rubin, R. T., & Poland, R. E. (1983). Neuroendocrine function in depression. In J. Angst (Ed.), *The Origins of depression: Current concepts and approaches* (pp. 205–220). New York: Springer-Verlag.

Rubin, R. T., & Poland, R. E. (1984). The dexamethasone suppression test in depression: Advantages and limitations. In G. D. Burrows, T. R. Norman, & K. P. Maguire (Eds.), *Biological psychiatry: Recent studies* (pp. 76–83). London: John Libbey.

Rubin, R. T., Poland, R. E., & Lesser, I. M. (1989). Neuroendocrine aspects of primary endogenous depression: VIII. Pituitary-gonadal axis activity in male patients and matched control subjects. *Psychoneuroendocrinology, 14*, 217–229.

Rubin, R. T., Poland, R. E., & Lesser, I. M. (1990). Neuroendocrine aspects of primary endogenous depression: X. Serum growth hormone measures in patients and matched control subjects. *Biological Psychiatry, 27*, 1065–1082.

Rubin, R. T., Poland, R. E., Lesser, I. M., & Martin, D. J. (1987). Neuroendocrine aspects of primary endogenous depression: IV. Pituitary-thyroid axis activity in patients and matched control subjects. *Psychoneuroendocrinology, 12*, 333–347.

Rubin, R. T., Poland, R. E., Lesser, I. M., & Martin, D. J. (1989). Neuroendocrine aspects of primary endogenous depression: V. Serum prolactin measures in patients and matched control subjects. *Biological Psychiatry, 25*, 4–21.

Rubin, R. T., Poland, R. E., Lesser, I. M., Martin, D. J., Blodgett, A. L. N., & Winston, R. A. (1987). Neuroendocrine aspects of primary endogenous depression. III. Cortisol secretion in relation to diagnosis and symptom patterns. *Psychological Medicine, 17*, 609–619.

Rubin, R. T., Poland, R. E., Lesser, I. M., Winston, R. A., & Blodgett, A. L. N. (1987). Neuroendocrine aspects of primary endogenous depression: I. Cortisol secretory dynamics in patients and matched control subjects. *Archives of General Psychiatry, 44*, 329–336.

Sachar, E. J. (1975). Neuroendocrine abnormalities in depressive illness. In E. J. Sachar (Ed.), *Topics in psychoendocrinology* (pp. 135–156). New York: Grune and Stratton.

Schildkraut, J. J. (1965). The catecholamine hypothesis of affective disorders: A review of supporting evidence. *American Journal of Psychiatry, 122,* 509–522.

Selye, H. (1973). The evolution of the stress concept. *American Scientist, 61,* 692–699.

Siever, L. J., & Davis, K. L. (1985). Overview: Toward a dysregulation hypothesis of depression. *American Journal of Psychiatry, 142,* 1017–1031.

Siever, L. J., Uhde, T. W., Jimerson, D. C., Post, R. M., Lake, C. R., & Murphy, D. L. (1984). Differential inhibitory noradrenergic responses to clonidine in 25 depressed patients and 25 normal control subjects. *American Journal of Psychiatry, 141,* 733–741.

Siever, L., Uhde, T., Silberman, E., Jimerson, D., Aloi, A., Post, R., & Murphy, D. (1982). Growth hormone response to clonidine as a probe of noradrenergic receptor responsiveness in affective disorder patients and controls. *Psychiatry Research, 6,* 171–183.

Spitzer, R. L., Endicott, J., & Robins, E. (1978). Research diagnostic criteria: Rationale and reliability. *Archives of General Psychiatry, 35,* 773–782.

Stanley, M., & Mann, J. J. (1983). Serotonin-2 binding sites are increased in the frontal cortex of suicide victims. *Lancet*: i: 214–216.

Swerdlow, N. R., & Koob, G. F. (1987). Dopamine, schizophrenia, mania, and depression: Toward a unified hypothesis of cortico-striato-pallido-thalamic function. *Behavioral and Brain Sciences, 10,* 197–243.

Träskman, L., Tybring, G., Åsberg, M., Bertillson, L., Lantto, O., & Schalling, D. (1980). Cortisol in the CSF of depressed and suicidal patients. *Archives of General Psychiatry, 37,* 761–767.

Tuomisto, J., & Männistö, P. (1985). Neurotransmitter regulation of anterior pituitary hormones. *Pharmacological Reviews, 37,* 249–332.

VanLoon, G. R. (1973). Brain catecholamines and ACTH secretion. In W. F. Ganong & L. Martini, (Eds.), *Frontiers in neuroendocrinology 1973* (pp. 209–247). New York: Oxford University Press.

Weiner, R. I., & Ganong, W. F. (1978). Role of brain monoamines and histamine in regulation of anterior pituitary secretion. *Physiological Reviews, 38,* 905–976.

Zimmerman, M., & Spitzer, R. L. (1989). Melancholia: From DSM-III to DSM-III-R. *American Journal of Psychiatry, 146,* 20–28.

# CHAPTER 3

# Can Coping and Competence Override Stress and Vulnerability in Schizophrenia?

*Sally Joy MacKain, Robert Paul Liberman, and Patrick W. Corrigan*

A MONG the most prominent and challenging features of schizophrenia is the vast intra- and interindividual variability of the course and outcome of the illness. A person with schizophrenia is seldom suffering from the symptoms of the illness 24 hours a day, 7 days a week. Likewise, one person with a diagnosis of schizophrenia may have a single occurrence of the illness and then return to a fairly normal level of functioning, while another individual may develop a recurrent pattern of hospital admissions and discharges, with a chronic, downhill course.

Heterogeneity in the phenomenology of schizophrenia may reflect the presence of a group of underlying disorders. Variations among and within individuals also can be explained by a model of a single illness influenced by stress, vulnerability, and protective factors. In this multidimensional model, enduring and genetically mediated psychobiological abnormalities yield an increased vulnerability to stressors, which give rise to diverse constellations of symptom impairments, associated social and vocational disabilities, and handicaps in role functioning (Liberman, 1986). Protective factors, such as antipsychotic medication, premorbid social competence, and supportive family environments can mitigate the noxious effects of vulnerability and stressors. An important goal of psychosocial rehabilitation is to increase patients' repertoires of instrumental and interpersonal skills to improve their ability to cope with a stressful world. Through acquiring and using coping skills, the likelihood of stress-induced relapse is diminished.

What skills are important as protective factors, and how are the skills taught most effectively? What factors affect the durability and generalizability of coping skills, and do these skills actually reduce patients' vulnera-

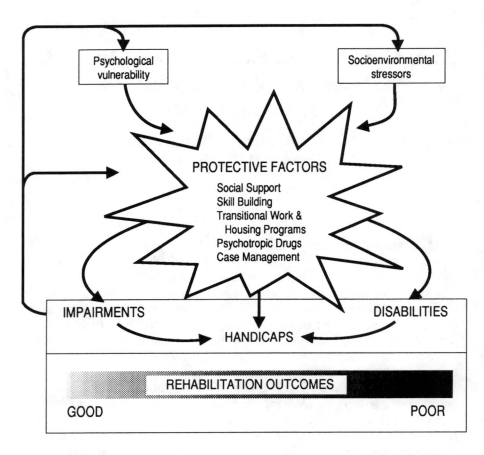

**FIGURE 3.1** In the stress–vulnerability–protective factors model of schizophrenia, the noxious effects of socioenvironmental stressors, superimposed on psychobiological vulnerability, can be buffered or mitigated by protective factors such as social support, antipsychotic medication, and skills training. The enormous variability in these three domains of variables accounts for the great heterogeneity in the course and outcome of schizophrenic disorders.

bility to succumbing to future stress? As depicted in Figure 3.1, does an improved repertoire of interpersonal and instrumental skills, combined with medication and social support, counterbalance stress superimposed on vulnerability? Do social skills translate into a scenario where patients' quality of life is really enhanced? In this chapter, we describe how the stress-vulnerability-protective model of schizophrenia may account for the striking variability of the illness. We focus on skills training as a means of improving the coping and competence among those diagnosed with schizophrenia.

# THE STRESS-VULNERABILITY-PROTECTIVE MODEL

The stress-vulnerability-protective model integrates physiological and behavioral aspects of schizophrenia (Nuechterlein & Dawson, 1984; Zubin & Spring, 1977). As a result of presumed genetic anomalies (Gottesman, McGuffin, & Farmer, 1987), in utero teratogens (Torrey, 1988), perinatal injury (Mednick et al., 1988), or infancy pandysmaturation (Fish, 1987), schizophrenics develop a range of psychophysiological and cognitive deficits that typically emerge in subclinical form during childhood, adolescence, or young adulthood. Limits in functioning have been identified in sustained attention (Nuechterlein, 1977), iconic memory (Sacuzzo, 1986), long term recall (Koh, 1978), response selection (Broen, 1968) and executive functioning (Weinberger, Berman, & Zec, 1986; Weinberger, BErman, & Illowsky, 1988). Skin conductance, heart rate, and blood pressure findings suggest that people with schizophrenia suffer from aberrant arousal patterns, which may contribute to a higher sensitivity to stressors (Gjerde, 1983). Even when impairments, disabilities, and handicaps are not present, as during premorbid and remission periods, these abnormalities persist and lead to an afflicted person's vulnerability to stressors.

Superimposed on vulnerability are physicochemical and social stressors such as street drugs and alcohol, comorbidity of physical illnesses, overstimulating environments, and emotionally intrusive relationships in treatment, residential, and family settings. Relapse is closely associated with stressful life experiences in the weeks prior to symptom exacerbation (Birley & Brown, 1970; Brown, Harris, & Peto, 1973; Lukoff, Snyder, Ventura, & Nuechterlein, 1984; Ventura, Nuechterlein, & Mintz, 1991). Furthermore, low tolerance for stress and episodes of acute symptomatology combine in reverberating cycles to increase the frequency and severity of stressful life events in the future. Compounding vulnerability are poor cognitive abilities which may preclude the susceptible person's acquisition of social and coping skills during the prodromal years. Considering the interactions between the many forms of stressors and enduring psychobiological vulnerability, it is not surprising that the course and outcome of schizophrenia varies so greatly among and within individuals.

Stress and vulnerability may be filtered and buffered through certain protective factors, such as coping skills, social support systems, and psychotropic drugs (Liberman, Nuechterlein, & Wallace, 1982). These "stress buffers" do not altogether prevent relapse, but rather reduce the probability that the noxious combination of stress and vulnerability will result in morbid outcomes.

For example, Emily, a 39-year-old woman with schizophrenia, has a part-time job at the public library, where she has established a warmly supportive set of relationships with her supervisor and co-workers. She visits her sister and family on the weekends and enjoys the benefits of a caring and affirming emotional climate. She is able to converse on a variety of subjects with verve and curiosity. She has been seeing the same psychiatrist for 10 years and has been educated by him in the benefits and side effects of antipsychotic medication. She is compliant with her medication regimen with the encouragement of her psychiatrist, and is able to monitor warning signs of stress and impending relapse and obtain early intervention when her stress indicators flare up. Twice in the past 5 years she has noticed increases in suspiciousness and the onset of insomnia, and both times has been benefitted by time-limited increases in therapy visits and doses of her neuroleptic medication. Her symptoms are in remission, although she continues to live a life of rather limited social contacts and activities. She has lived continuously in the community for 8 years, without need for hospitalization. She has consistently taken her prescribed medication and has a number of friends in the apartment building where she lives. For this woman, the stress and vulnerability remain fairly evenly balanced, through the help of a number of protective factors, such as the social support and effective coping skills required for living independently.

Unfortunately, protective factors may not be available to many schizophrenic individuals who, because of the volatile course of the disease, often become estranged from family members, friends, and co-workers. A typical example of a person for whom stress and vulnerability outweigh protective factors is Les, a 21-year-old man who has been admitted to a psychiatric facility for the third time in one year. Les has lost a number of jobs due to absences and difficulty getting along with his supervisors, has had no contact with his family in 9 months, and has no friends. He also abuses alcohol, which ultimately sabotages the protective effects of psychotropic medication. Likewise, Les's isolation from friends and family deprive him of opportunities to gain the social and emotional support he so clearly needs.

Through psychoeducational methods of rehabilitation, individuals with schizophrenia can strengthen social and instrumental skills that can increase their ability to cope with daily stressors, buffer their biological vulnerabilities, and broaden their social support networks. In support of this model, drug and psychosocial treatment have been found to have synergistic effects (Falloon & Liberman, 1983a; Liberman, Corrigan, & Schade, 1989). In conjunction with judicious drug therapy, skills training has been found in a growing number of studies to improve symptomatology and reduce relapse rates (e.g., Bellack, Turner, Hersen, & Luber, 1984; Hogarty et al., 1986; Paul & Lentz, 1977; Wallace & Liberman, 1985). Patients who receive skills training may eventually require lower dosages of antipsychotic medications than patients who do not (Falloon, 1985; Wirshing, Eckman, Liberman, & Marder, 1990). Both longitudinal, naturalistic, and more controlled treatment studies validate the importance of insulating the vulnerable individual from stress through a blending of protective factors such as medication, social support, and skills training. The remainder of this chapter will focus on the forms, mode, generalizability, durability, and benefits of skills training as one of the most protective factors in treating schizophrenia.

## IDENTIFYING ESSENTIAL SKILLS

In which skills should individuals and families receive training to enable them to cope with stress and vulnerability? First, a functional assessment should be conducted to specify individualized treatment goals (Kuehnel, 1988; Wallace, 1986). For example, treatment goals for Les, the young man described above, might include learning how to monitor and manage side effects of his prescribed antipsychotic medications; improving eye contact and lowering voice volume so he can communicate more effectively; and learning more about how alcohol adversely affects his physical and mental health.

If patients and caregivers are to counteract stress and vulnerability effectively, a number of behavioral competencies must be targeted, such as management of medications and symptoms, improving personal hygiene, productive use of leisure time, locating and maintaining employment, problem solving, conversation skills, money management, and food preparation. While this list is by no means exhaustive, it covers many of the basic needs and skills related to successful adaptation to the community and a fulfilling life.

Once goals have been identified, the procedures used must be appropriately structured to meet the attentional and cognitive limitations particular to the schizophrenic individual. Ideally, however, the teaching strategy must also be flexible enough to be adapted to a variety of settings and used with patients of diverse levels of functioning.

## THE NATURE OF SKILLS TRAINING

Skills training utilizes procedures based on basic principles of human learning to train in specific independent living and interpersonal skills and to promote generalization and maintenance of these skills. While many psychosocial treatment programs claim to do skills training, nonspecific group activities that engage patients in "socialization" should be distinguished from methods which systematically use social and behavioral learning techniques in a structured approach to skills building (Liberman, DeRisi, & Mueser, 1989; Liberman, Mueser, Wallace, Jacobs, Eckman, & Massel, 1986).

A skills training approach differs from other, less specific approaches that target "socialization" in that skills training techniques are highly structured, directive, and based on principles of operant and social learning theory. In accordance with operant principles, individuals who emit behaviors in response to situational stimuli are more likely to show the behavior in similar, future situations if the behavior is reinforced (Skinner, 1953). According to social learning theory, individuals are likely to acquire a behavior by watching a model perform it correctly, especially if the model is subsequently reinforced in that performance (Bandura, 1969). These principles are the "heart and soul" of skills training procedures, which include instructions, modeling, behavioral rehearsal, feedback, contingent reinforcement, and homework (Liberman, DeRisi, & Mueser, 1989).

Similar procedures are used by teachers in every classroom, from kindergarten to graduate school, and by trainers in industrial, office, and service settings. However, people with schizophrenia typically have "learning disabilities", or attentional and memory deficits imposed by their illness (Andreasen, 1982; Nuechterlein & Dawson, 1984). Therefore, information must be made even more explicit, and presented with more repetition and through a variety of media that encourages learning by "seeing," "hearing," and "doing." To combat negative symptoms such as amotivation, social withdrawal, and poverty of speech, trainers providing this "special education" provide specific, genuine praise for even the slightest improvements in effort and skill. In addition, the structure, practicality, and predictability of skills training procedures can help compensate for intellectual impairments associated with schizophrenia, such as poor memory and concentration (Liberman, 1988).

An innovative approach to teaching social and independent living skills to seriously mentally ill people has been developed at the UCLA Clinical Research Center for Schizophrenia and Psychiatric Rehabilitation, cosponsored by the Brentwood/Los Angeles VA Medical Center, and Camarillo State Hospital. Drs. Robert Liberman and Charles Wallace and their colleagues have incorporated learning principles and training methods in the production of a highly structured, modular approach to skills training. Training models that have been developed so far include *Medication Management, Symptom Management, Recreation for Leisure, Basic Conversation Skills,* and *Grooming and Personal Hygiene* (Liberman & Corrigan, 1991). Each module represents a structured curriculum and consists of a trainer's manual that prescribes specifically what is to be done and said during any given lesson, a patients' workbook that contains various fact sheets and checklists, and a demonstration video that models the skills to be taught.

The *content* of each module is divided into four to eight skill areas. For example, the *Medication Management* module contains five skill areas: 1) Obtaining information about antipsychotic medication; 2) Knowing correct self-administration and evaluation of medication; 3) Identifying and managing side effects of medication; 4) Negotiating medication issues with health care providers; and 5) Using long-acting injectable medication.

Although the *content* of the modules differs, the *process* by which each skill area of each module is taught remains constant. The same seven learning activities, or learning steps, appear in every skill area of every module:

1) Introduction to the Skill Area. The trainer defines key terms and encourages group members to identify ways in which learning the skills might benefit them. This builds motivation in patients. For example, in the introduction to the first skill area of the *Symptom Self Management* module, participants are asked: "How will a better understanding of your illness improve the quality of your life?"

2) Videotape Questions and Answers. Videotaped actors model a set of target behaviors successfully. The trainer pauses the tape periodically to ask the group members specified questions to increase patient involve-

ment and to assess comprehension. In the *Basic Conversation Skills* module, for instance, skill area 3 teaches participants how to keep a friendly conversation going. The videotape for this section shows actors using verbal active listening behaviors, asking open- and closed-ended questions, identifying new topics, and making self-disclosing statements.

3) Roleplay Exercises. Participants are given the opportunity to practice the skills they have recently viewed on the video, and to learn effective communication skills. Group members are encouraged to repeat their role-plays until they can demonstrate that they have learned the information and skills demonstrated earlier on the video. The group leader or trainer, using shaping and modeling techniques, may choose to videotape roleplays and offer specific, positive feedback to the participant as the video is replayed. Participants in the *Medication Management* module, for example, practice communicating concerns about medication side effects with their psychiatrists.

4) Resource Management. Participants learn to identify and obtain resources essential to the skill being learned; for example, in the *Medication Management* module, the money and transportation required to get to the doctor for information about medication.

5) Outcome Problems. Participants learn a seven-step method for solving problems that may arise when trying to use the skill. For example, in the *Recreation for Leisure* module, participants in skill area 4 (evaluating a recreational activity) tackle the problem of wanting to continue a recreational activity but not being able to afford a needed piece of equipment.

6) In Vivo Exercises. Participants practice the newly learned skills in situations outside the training environment; the trainer accompanies the patient to provide moral support, prompts, and feedback. In skill area 1 of the *Medication Management* module (obtaining information about medication), the trainer sits in on a patient's appointment with the psychiatrist while the patient asks questions about his/her medication.

7) Homework Exercises. Group members perform the skill in a "real life" situation without trainer support; for example, in the *Basic Conversations Skills* module, participants observe two other people having a pleasant conversation and complete a worksheet on the use of active verbal listening skills.

Each learning step builds on information learned in previous steps, and takes into consideration the cognitive characteristics of people with serious mental illness. For example, information is presented in brief "chunks" using multimedia aids and both auditory and visual input channels, and is repeated in different ways throughout a module to help compensate for the attention and memory difficulties often associated with chronic psychiatric disabilities.

The first three learning activities, *Introduction, Videotape*, and *Roleplay*, focus on skill acquisition and are conducted within a treatment or classroom setting. The remaining activities are intended to promote generalization of skills acquired in therapeutic environments. The problem solving techniques embedded in the fourth and fifth learning activities, *Resource Management* and *Outcome Problems*, occur in a treatment setting, but involve anticipation of obstacles the patient might encounter in the future, when attempting to implement the skill in "real life." The two final learning activities, *In Vivo* and *Homework*, are also directed at improving the transfer of skills and take place in the patient's natural environment. Patients who are able to complete the homework exercise "pass" the learning criteria for that particular skill area of a module. Group leaders are encouraged to conduct "booster sessions" periodically after a module has been completed to review material and help participants keep their skills polished.

There are a number of advantages to packaging social skills training into a modular format. First, the prescriptive format is "user friendly," so that paraprofessionals, such as residential care facility staff, who most frequently assume direct care of the chronically mentally ill (Graziano & Katz, 1982), can use the materials effectively. The structured, "cookbook" approach of the trainer's manuals means that minimal effort is required to plan and conduct the sessions each day, and trainers can easily substitute for one another. Methods for documenting participants' progress are built into the module. Pretests and posttests are included in the patient workbooks, and trainers are provided with progress checklists for ease of tracking trainees' performances and participation. These resources greatly assist in quality assurance, program evaluation, and treatment outcome research. Additionally, the consistency with which the modules can be implemented in a variety of settings means that individuals can begin a module as inpatients and continue their training on an outpatient basis at a day treatment center or residential care facility.

## CAN SCHIZOPHRENICS LEARN SOCIAL AND INDEPENDENT LIVING SKILLS?

Evidence for the effectiveness of skills training comes from a number of studies. A meta-analysis of two dozen publications assessed effects of social skills training along the dimensions of skill acquisition, generalization of skills to other settings or behaviors, social adjustment, relapse, and reduction of psychotic symptoms, this study found statistically significant effect sizes for treatment versus control groups (Benton & Schroeder, 1990).

For example, social and conversational skills training delivered in fourteen 90-minute training sessions for seven long-stay, mixed diagnosis female residents of a token economy ward resulted in increased eye contact, better posture, less psychotic talk, and improved general conversational ability (Fecteau & Duffy, 1986). Likewise, in another study, 28 male chronic schizophrenic patients were randomly assigned to either a life skills training program or to a control condition (Brown & Munford, 1983). Patients in both groups received 20 hours of programmed treatment activities per week for 3 months. The skills training program focused on interpersonal skills, nutrition, health, personal finances, time management, and community networking skills. Change scores on self-report measures and role-play assessments indicated that individuals in the training program successfully learned skills in these areas.

Some skills training programs focus on the acquisition of cognitive skills in addition to overt behaviors. For example, training curricula have been designed to target social perception and cognitive self-management skills (Van Dam-Baggen & Kraaimaat, 1986), problem solving (Donahoe, Carter, Bloen, Hirsch, Laasi, & Wallace, 1990; Hansen, St. Lawrence, & Christoff, 1985; Sullivan, Marder, Liberman, Donahoe, & Mintz, 1990), and information processing skills (Wallace, 1982). Wallace and Liberman (1985) reported the results of a controlled trial of social skills training for 28 male schizophrenic patients. The patients were randomly assigned to either an intensive social skills training program or to an equally intensive "holistic health therapy" program. Skills training focused on "receiving" and "processing" components of interpersonal problem solving skills, as well as "sending" appropriate responses. In addition, patients assigned to this program received behavioral family therapy which emphasized training in communication and problem solving skills. "Holistic health therapy" focused on coping with life stressors through the use of yoga, meditation, walking, and jogging. Patients in this treatment group received supportive, insight-oriented family therapy. Patients in both programs received 6 hours of scheduled treatment daily for 9 weeks. Results showed that only individuals in the skills training program acquired receiving and processing skills, based on their improved performance on questions designed to assess their ability to attend to and accurately perceive problem situations, to interpret interpersonal cues, and to generate, evaluate, and select reasonable response alternatives. The holistic approach may be effective in conjunction with skills training, but did not promote development of community adaptation skills on its own.

The Social and Independent Living Skills modules developed at UCLA have been field tested extensively at state hospitals, residential treatment facilities, and community mental health centers around the country. Results of the field tests indicate that 1) participants significantly improved their knowledge and performance of the skills taught in the modules; 2) staff accurately and easily implemented the modules with a minimum of training; and 3) both staff and patients experienced positive effects that extended beyond acquisition of the skills; participants' attentiveness and responsiveness increased both in and out of the training sessions (Wallace, Liberman, MacKain, Blackwell, & Eckman, 1993). The efficacy of these modules in improving patient knowledge and social and independent living skills has also been tested and documented in schizophrenics receiving treatment at a VA hospital and state prison (i.e., MacKain & Streveler, 1990; Wirshing et al., 1990).

While the research literature suggests that skills training aids the acquisition of basic coping skills and competencies, methodological problems must be addressed in future research. For example, the validity of dependent measures used to assess the acquisition of skills is limited. Particularly worthy of further investigation is the use of role-played "performances" as evidence that a skill has been learned, when support for a relationship between role-played behavior and spontaneous occurrences of that behavior in natural environments is decidedly weak (Bellack, Hersen, & Lamparski, 1979; Bellack, Hersen, & Turner, 1976; Kazdin, Matson, & Esveldt-Dawson, 1984). Naturalistic observation of target behaviors would be a more valid method of assessment, but raises ethical questions and is time-consuming and expensive (Morrison, 1990).

Similarly, the evaluation of skills acquired by psychiatric patients continues to be limited by the lack of data on competent social behavior in normal individuals (Morrison & Bellack, 1987). Limited information is available regarding specific components of skilled complex social functioning, making identification of those skill components which are most relevant to normal functioning difficult. Nevertheless, numerous controlled studies indicate that severely mentally ill individuals can indeed acquire information and specified skills related to coping and adaptation.

## ARE THE ACQUIRED SKILLS DURABLE AND GENERALIZABLE

Ultimately, the best test of the efficacy of skills training is whether the skills last and are actually used and applied in other settings and situations. In their meta-analysis, Benton and Schroeder (1990) concluded that durability and generalization of skills training effects were measured less frequently than basic skill acquisition and, when they were assessed, were found to occur but not as robustly as training effects on skills acquisition.

## Durability

Evidence regarding the durability of social and life skills has largely been positive when training has been sufficiently intensive, long-term, and comprehensive, Several studies have shown that acquired skills are still performed at adequate levels 1–3 months later (Brown, 1982; Frisch, El-liot, Atsaides, Salva, & Denney, 1982; Jaffe & Carlson, 1976; Wallace, Boone, Donahoe, & Foy, 1985) Other studies have shown that skills can be maintained over much longer periods (Holmes, Hansen, & St. Lawrence, 1984; Liberman, Mueser, Wallace, Jacobs, et al., 1986; Monti, Curran, Corriveau, & DeLancey, 1980; Wallace et al., 1993) with two studies demonstrating that skills were reported at significant levels two years after training (Kindness & Newton, 1984; Longin & Rooney, 1975). Contradictory evidence from two studies shows that skills were not maintained after 2–3 months had passed (Spencer, Gillespie, & Ekisa, 1983; Van Dam-Baggen & Kraaimaat, 1986), but these studies did not employ intensive training with overlearning.

Few studies include follow-up data, due to the complexities involved in locating and assessing psychiatric patients over long periods of time. Those follow-up studies that do exist have received the same criticisms of most studies of skill acquisition: that durability of an acquired skill tends to be measured by role-play and information/interview tests, despite the questionable validity and reliability of these methods.

## Generalizability

Numerous investigators have been able to demonstrate that acquired skills can transfer to different situations (Falloon, Lindley, MacDonald, & Marks, 1977; Goldsmith & McFall, 1975; Hersen, Eisler, & Miller, 1974; Kazdin, 1974; Liberman, Mueser, & Wallace, 1986; McFall & Lil-lesand, 1971). Results of a recent study on problemsolving suggest that improved identification of problem components and increased generation of relevant solutions may generalize to related interpersonal behaviors (Hansen et al., 1985). These investigators found that seven chronically disabled individuals were able to broaden their repertoires of responses to a variety of problem situations.

The use of intensively applied, cognitively oriented skills training techniques has yielded better generalization of skills to new situations. For example, a cohort of schizophrenics at high risk for relapse received 30 hours per week of social skills training that focused on teaching patients to actively "solve" their problems (Wallace & Liberman, 1985). Results showed improvement not only in targeted skills, but also in domains of social functioning that were not trained. Similarly, in a study of skills training within the family context, Falloon (1985) found that weekly, biweekly, then monthly training sessions over a 2-year period resulted in generalized improvements in employment, friendships, and functioning within the home.

Participants in field testing of the Social and Independent Living Skills modules commented that the modules gave them valuable skills and information that generalized to their daily lives (Blair & Wallace, 1989; MacKain & Wallace, 1988; Wallace et al., 1993). Several participants in the *Recreation for Leisure* module continued for at least a year to engage in activities they had learned and practiced during the training. Others in the *Medication Management* module described improved communication with their physicians, and staff reported improved medication compliance and fewer complaints among residents who had been randomly assigned to participate (Eckman, Liberman, Blair, & Phipps, 1990).

On the other hand, limited generalization of social skills training among the seriously mentally ill has been reported by a number of researchers and clinicians (Kazdin & Bootzin, 1972; Wallace, 1976). Several studies have found that acquired behaviors did not transfer to other settings (Cole, Klarreich, & Fryatt, 1982; Frederiksen, Jenkins, Foy, & Eisler, 1976; Hersen et al., 1974). Typically, assessment of generalization has focused on whether functioning within independent domains such as work or recreation has improved. Early findings in this area were largely negative (Bellack, Hersen, & Turner, 1976; Hersen, Eisler, & Miller, 1973; McFall & Lillesand, 1971; McFall & Twentyman, 1971). It should be pointed out, however, that these earlier studies implemented relatively brief programs of social skills training which, in retrospect, would not have been sufficient to produce durable and generalizable outcomes.

Future research efforts should be directed toward accounting for the divergence in findings to response and stimulus generalization and identifying relationships between specific treatment variables and outcome. Conflicting results may be attributed to differences in diagnostic procedures, medication status, severity of psychopathology, training procedures, assessment methods, or differences in the criterion used to determine whether or not generalization has taken place. Despite these caveats, recent research using better designed techniques of social skills training do suggest that acquired skills can be maintained for relatively long periods, at least based on role-play tests of knowledge and skill performance. More work needs to be done on evaluating generalization of skills to other settings, situations, and behaviors before the efficacy of any single approach over another can be verified.

# DOES AN INCREASED REPERTOIRE OF SKILLS LEAD TO DIMINISHED SYMPTOMS AND ENHANCED QUALITY OF LIFE

A major goal of social skills training is to improve the patient's ability to function effectively in real-life settings. Beyond improvement in role functioning, successful training should also be associated with reductions in the frequency and severity of psychiatric symptoms, thereby helping to reduce relapse rates and rehospitalization. Ideally, skills acquired through training will protect an individual against relapse by strengthening his or her ability to cope with stressors and challenges from the natural environment.

## Symptom Reduction

A meta-analysis of studies involving skills training for chronically mentally ill individuals suggested that comprehensive social skills training reduces clinical symptoms in psychiatric patients, although the effects were less than for the acquisition of skills (Benton & Schroeder, 1990). Among schizophrenic inpatients and outpatients who are stabilized on medication, intensive social skills training significantly lowered symptoms (Falloon, Boyd, McGill, Razani, Moss, & Gilderman, 1982; Liberman, Falloon, & Wallace, 1984; Wallace & Liberman, 1985). Similarly, schizophrenics who participated in a day hospital program and received social skills training showed more durable symptom reductions over a 6-month follow-up period than did patients in the same program who did not receive skills training (Bellack et al., 1984). In depressed outpatients, skills training has been found to have clinical effects equivalent to antidepressant medication, and has been associated with a lower rate of dropout from treatment than medication alone or cognitive therapy (Bellack, Hersen, & Himmelhoch, 1983; Miller, Norman, & Keitner, 1989).

Hogarty and his colleagues (Hogarty et al., 1986) determined the effects of psychosocial treatment on preventing or postponing exacerbation of psychiatric symptoms by following 90 schizophrenic and schizoaffective patients at high risk for relapse. Relapse was defined as a change from "nonpsychotic" status at discharge to "psychotic" status. Examination of relapse rates in the total sample 12 months after treatment indicated that both behavioral family therapy and social skills training were associated with lower relapse rates. While 41% of the patients in the medication-alone group relapsed during the year-long followup period, only about 20% of those patients assigned to either family therapy or to skills training experienced relapse. *None* of the patients who received both family therapy and skills training relapsed. Moreover, data from a subsample of verifiably drug-compliant individuals revealed a similar pattern of results, indicating that these psychosocial interventions exerted therapeutic effects over and above the protective effects of medication.

Medication compliance plays a central role in mitigating symptom exacerbation and relapse in schizophrenia (Donaldson, Gelenberg, & Galdessarni, 1983). For this reason, creators of the *Medication Management* module aimed to teach patients to become more reliable, informed, and responsible consumers of maintenance antipsychotic drugs (Eckman, Liberman, Blair, & Phipps, 1990; Wallace, 1988). Additionally, it was hypothesized that patients who would learn skills taught in the *Symptom Self-Management* module should experience a reduction in relapse and rehospitalization rates, since they would be able to identify warning signs of an impending relapse and seek early intervention. These hypotheses are currently being researched more systematically in three NIMH- and VA-supported controlled studies at the UCLA Clinical Research Center for Schizophrenia and Psychiatric Rehabilitation.

Recent data on social skills training and psychiatric symptom relapse are encouraging, and indicate that skills training programs place patients at lowered risk for relapse. However, relapse rates differ from study to study, and may fluctuate depending on a number of factors, including the stage or severity of the mental disorder and the lack of comparable definitions of relapse. The length of the follow-up period is also critical. Skills training programs demonstrate greater relapse-prevention effects within a year after treatment. Relapse rates increase over time, with longer follow-up periods. This suggests that social skills training programs effectively delay, rather than prevent, major exacerbations of psychiatric symptoms (Hogarty et al., 1986; Hogarty, Anderson, & Reiss, 1987). However, since a goal of rehabilitation is to help provide coping skills to protect the highly sensitive person from stressors, extended skills training, with "brush-up sessions" and continued social support, case management, and reinforcement, may allow the patient to counterbalance stress and vulnerability effectively.

## Quality of Life

Despite research documenting that social skills training improves social competence and decreases symptoms, few studies have investigated whether this technology improves patient satisfaction with day-to-day living. Liberman et al. (1986) measured this construct using Strauss and Carpenter's (1972, 1974) criteria before and after social skills training. Results showed that patients' everyday lives improved in two areas: 1) positive symptoms significantly diminished; while 2) employment activity improved. In the same study, families rated their schizophrenic young adult offspring on several domains using the Katz Adjustment Scales, Revised (Wallace & Liberman, 1985). In contrast with the control group, the relatives of patients who received social skills training reported more satisfaction with the activities of their adult offspring who were now busier with church, friends, family, and leisure activities. However, the skills training program was confounded by concurrent behavioral family therapy; thus improved ratings on the Katz may have represented more benevolent attitudes regarding the severely disabled family member as a result of increased knowledge about the disease.

Using a single-subject design, Marzillier and Winter (1978) sought an explanation for the lack of overall improvement in social adjustment for four subjects who had demonstrated clear gains in social skills in a treatment setting. They concluded that extratherapeutic change requires that skills training be but one component of a comprehensive approach. They subsequently provided relaxation and cognitive interventions for these individuals and found that overall functioning was enhanced. Their findings have been reaffirmed by others who have provided more comprehensive systems of care (Hogarty et al., 1986; Vaccaro & Liberman, 1989).

From a community perspective, social and independent living skills training indirectly improves quality of life to the extent that frequency and intensity of relapse can decrease. Hospital stays can thus be shortened, theoretically enabling patients to return to the community in which they enjoy the privileges society has to offer. Unfortunately, social skills training in particular, and community mental health in general, has yet to reach its full potential (Bellack & Mueser, 1986). A majority of chronically mentally ill individuals who reside in urban environments and receive outpatient care have marginal lives at best (Klerman, 1977; Lehman, Ward, & Linn, 1982).

# IMPORTANCE OF INCORPORATING SKILLS TRAINING INTO THE PATIENT'S NATURAL SOCIAL ECOLOGY

Given the plight of the severely disabled outpatient, improvement of community applications of skills training is clearly indicated. Future research on the effect of skills training on quality of life must include evaluations of the social system in which training occurs and in which the patient will be placed (Shepherd, 1986). Also, to maximize the probability that the effects of skills training will last and be generalized to other settings, situations, and behaviors, mental health professionals must constantly try to incorporate the patient's natural environment into the training. Most often, skills training takes place in a classroom or other artificial setting. While staff might rejoice at a patient's improvements in skill performance in the training room, the crucial question is, "Will he use it outside the classroom, where it really counts?"

The patient's world—her present and future settings and situations—is ever changing and difficult to characterize. Yet, that world must be simultaneously incorporated into three aspects of the patient's treatment. First, the *content* of the training must be relevant to the patient's social ecology; second, the *process* of the training should involve overt programming for generalization to current and future (e.g., post-discharge) settings and situations; and finally, treatment efforts undertaken within the patient's larger community must be *comprehensive, consistent,* and *coordinated*.

## Content Relevance

Every effort should be made to thoroughly specify the intended goals for treatment. For example, it sounds simple enough to teach an individual how to communicate needs to a caregiver or roommate. However, failure to consider the specific settings, people, personalities, situations, and obstacles that may await the patient outside the training room will severely restrict any positive effects of training. Since generalization requires that the individual use the skill when and where it counts most—at home, in one's own room, at work, with family, peers, doctors, and employers—the skills trainer should attempt to incorporate information about the patient's current setting and about the setting to which the patient will be discharged. As such, the trainer must bring in the "real world" and incorporate it into the skills training.

The seriously mentally ill prison inmate represents a dramatic example of a skills training situation in which "bringing in" the real world is particularly important. A schizophrenic inmate who has difficulty expressing feelings and needs may be appropriately placed in a social skills training group that emphasizes assertive behavior and freer expression of emotions. The inmate may become highly skilled in communicating his needs and feelings to others. Outside the training room, however, in the general prison facility, expression of feelings may be interpreted as a sign of weakness, making him even more vulnerable to other inmates who may take advantage of him. Moreover, communicating needs in an assertive way may be adaptive when relating to family or friends, but can be interpreted as aggression or resistance if directed at correctional personnel (MacKain & Streveler, 1990).

While assertive communication and expression of feelings in most contexts would promote coping and adaptation, in a prison, assertion could lead to disciplinary action or even physical harm. Although it is not always easy to anticipate the setting and situations a patient might face, failure to do so can sabotage the beneficial effects of treatment.

## Process: Programming for Generalization

"Bringing in" the natural, extratherapeutic environment by integrating it into the context of the training via the modification of content is the first step in promoting durability and generalization of skills taught. At the same time, efforts should be made to *bring out* the treatment, taking the skills-building activities into the patient's own world of circumstances and surroundings.

Another good example of this approach is family treatment that attempts to teach families ways to cope with and manage schizophrenic patients living at home. In their review of studies on the effectiveness of psychosocial family interventions, Tarrier and Barrowclough (1990) claim there is ample evidence to support behavioral family treatments in reducing relapse in patients living in high-risk environments. Behavioral Family

Management (BFM) (Falloon & Liberman, 1983b) involves teaching patients and their families about schizophrenia and trains them in problem-solving and communication skills. In a controlled study, the effectiveness of BFM as compared to individual therapy was evaluated in 36 young adult schizophrenics who were living at home in stressful, tense relationships with parents. Individuals were randomly assigned to receive BFM at home, or individual, supportive therapy in a clinic. After 9 months of treatment, only 6% of the patients receiving BFM had relapsed, while 44% of the subjects receiving individual therapy did so. After 2 years, relapse rates had increased, with 17% of BFM recipients and 83% of individual therapy clients experiencing relapse (Falloon et al., 1982; Falloon et al., 1985). In addition, overall social adjustment, recreational activity, family life, work, and family burden improved for the Behavioral Family Management group as well. These findings have recently been replicated (Randolph et al., 1993).

The procedures are behavioral in that principles of learning and behavior change are systematically employed (Liberman, 1986), and the training takes place within the context of the schizophrenic individual's "real world." Whether BFM occurs in the hospital, clinic, or home—an essential component of the patient's social ecology—his family is present.

It may be ideal to provide skills training in the patient's natural environment, but it is costly, time-consuming, and usually impractical. In most cases, patients are transported to a central location to receive skills training, such as a day-treatment center at a community mental health center, or an activities room within an inpatient setting. Given these practices, how can the training be "transported" into the patient's real world?

The Social and Independent Living Skills modules contain two learning activities designed to move the patient out from the training or therapy session and into the "world." The *In vivo* and *Homework* exercises are designed to occur with the patient's own physician, roommate, family, in the individual's own room, doctor's office, or home, whenever possible.

When actual relocation is not possible the trainer is encouraged to create a setting that approximates the settings and people associated with that individual. For example, a hospitalized patient may not be allowed to make a home visit to select an optimal place to store his medication. Instead, the patient's room can be simulated by arranging hospital furniture in configurations approximating his own room at the residential care facility in the community. The primary difference between the *In vivo* and *Homework* assignments is that the *Homework* assignments tend to be more challenging, since the trainer is not present to provide prompts or support.

Consequences of omitting these two learning activities are evident in the reports of several trainers who participated in the field testing of the Social and Independent Living Skills modules. In a controlled study, Wallace et al. (1993) found that patients at a large state hospital who completed a skills training program designed to teach grooming and personal hygiene were much more skilled in their role-plays and descriptions of the proper steps involved in bathing, shaving, hair care, and dental hygiene than were waiting list control subjects. However, neither the treatment nor control group improved in appearance or body odor. Trainers attributed the lack of change to the absence of *In vivo* and *Homework* exercises. All training occurred off the living units, in an "Achievement Center" without sinks or the patients' own grooming supplies. Because trainers did not have access to patients during their actual grooming time, early in the morning and late in the evening, *In vivo* and *Homework* exercises were skipped. Without opportunities to prompt and reinforce the trainees' grooming behaviors as they occurred naturally, the information and skills may not have transferred. Results from testing at other sites using the modules indicated that groups for whom the *In vivo* and *Homework* assignments were omitted showed less improvement in social skills than groups that participated in all seven learning activities (Corrigan, MacKain, & Liberman, in press; Blair & Wallace, 1989).

In a wide-scale effort to evaluate the potential to integrate skills training into residential care programs, board and care home operators throughout southern California received training in conducting the *Medication Management, Symptom Self-Management*, and *Recreation for Leisure* modules developed by Liberman and his colleagues. The quality of the training they provided to residents and the latter's acquisition of skills was evaluated. Results indicated that residential care staff, many with only a high school diploma, were at least as effective in teaching targeted skills as trainers with graduate degrees working in institutional settings.

Several residential care workers attributed their success in part to their many opportunities to observe residents in a variety of situations throughout the day: at meals, during free time, during morning grooming, and while doing assigned chores. Since they interacted with residents throughout the day, staff were able to provide reminders and praise for improvements. In providing skills training in a residential setting, staff are helping to maximize the chances that participants will use acquired skills in their daily lives. Staff also commented that residents became much more verbally supportive of each other in offering "compliments" for progress in a particular skill or for effort. Thus, even where staff is short-handed, residents receiving similar training can help reinforce learning among themselves in constructive ways.

## COORDINATED, CONTINUOUS, COMPREHENSIVE CARE

With the implementation of deinstitutionalization, many seriously mentally ill individuals are caught in the "revolving door" of relapse, rehospitalization, and relapse. Between 35–50% of chronically mentally ill patients who are discharged from hospitals are readmitted within 1 year (Anthony, Cohen, & Vitalo, 1978; Lamb, 1982). There has been renewed interest in the development of continuous care programs designed to link the hospitalized patient to a broader array of services available at community mental health centers and aftercare programs.

In a controlled study, Altman (1984) found that patients discharged into the community without prearranged aftercare appointments were three times more likely to be hospitalized within 1 year than were patients who had participated in an aftercare planning program. Yet, in actual practice, the term "aftercare" typically refers to psychiatric care offered at a community mental health center when the seriously mentally ill patient also needs help getting food, shelter, medical care, transportation, managing money, and finding and maintaining a job. Given that the provision of many of these services in the community tends to be so fragmented, researchers and clinicians have teamed up to reorganize provision of services to the chronically mentally ill and form intensive case management teams.

Borland and his colleagues (Borland, McRae, & Lycan, 1989) provided coordinated, intensive case management services to 72 young, treatment-resistant, chronically mentally ill patients continuously over a period of 5 years. Compared to baseline data gathered for 2 years before the study began, the number of days spent in the hospital was reduced by 75%. However, because the patients consumed more community-based services that were also expensive, net costs were not reduced under the intensive case management program.

Because of closer monitoring and more individualized assessment of patients' clinical needs, intensive case management can be expected to increase the utilization of treatment, rehabilitation and social services which should improve outcomes but not necessarily reduce costs. The best known system of intensive case management, called Training in Community Living, has been replicated in more than ten sites around the United States and Australia with impressive reduction in hospitalization rates and improvement in subjective quality of life (Test, 1992). However, these programs have not resulted in demonstrable improvements in social functioning, suggesting that the addition of systematic and structured social skills training methods might augment the benefits of intensive case management. When skills training has been added to the array of community-based services available to persons with schizophrenia, substantial improvements have been noted in social functioning and clinical outcome (Falloon & Fadden, 1993).

Integration of skills training with case management is much more likely to work when there is a uniform but flexible program, such as the Social and Independent Living Skills modules, that can be put in place at all jurisdictional levels. For example, while hospitalized, a patient may participate in a training group that teaches basic conversation skills using a very brief, simple modeling and role-play procedures. Next, she may progress to a more challenging group on assertion and also learn skills involved in medication management. After discharge, she could continue to receive training in these skills at the mental health center or in a group home. Training in other essential skills could be added, including self-management of symptoms and learning to use free time productively. The patient's case manager could work individually with her, for example, teaching her how to use public transportation, still using behavioral techniques of modeling, rehearsal, and practicing in vivo. The *process* of delivering services can be made more consistent, regardless of personnel and site changes, by reference to such a uniform training system.

Just as we build wheelchair ramps for the handicapped, so must we be willing to modify natural, social environments for chronically mentally ill individuals. For example, caregivers who come into contact with the patient should be sensitized to prompt and praise the mentally ill individual's coping efforts, to increase the possibility that the patient will use new social and life skills in his or her community. In this way, we not only incorporate elements of the natural environment in treatment settings, but also "program" the natural environment to support the results of training. This can be done by providing "booster sessions" to bolster the durability of the skills trained, as well as by guiding caregivers to offer daily reminders and positive reinforcement for even slight improvements.

## SUMMARY

Skills training, a highly structured approach based on operant and social learning principles, can serve as a buffer in the balance between stress and psychobiological vulnerability. With a solid background of skills training, patients may continue to be protected against relapse, perhaps with lower doses of medication. Even the most seriously mentally ill individuals can indeed learn social and independent living skills, but to be most effective the training must be intensive, long-term, and part of a larger, comprehensive treatment program so that the skills will last and be generalized to other situations, people, settings, and behaviors.

In addition, training must incorporate information about the patient's natural environment, be integrated into the patient's natural ecology whenever possible, and be consistently available regardless of the inevitable turnover in treatment staff. Finally, mentally ill persons' environments must also be modified, or "programmed," so that family members, roommates, counselors, and employers are sensitive to patients' vulnerability to stress and actively support their efforts to protect themselves from stress through the acquisition of coping skills and new competencies.

# REFERENCES

Altman, H. (1984). A collaborative approach to discharge planning for chronic mental patients. *Hospital and Community Psychiatry, 34,* 641–642.

Andreasen, N. C. (1982). Negative v. positive schizophrenia: Definition and validation. *Archives of General Psychiatry, 39,* 784–788.

Anderson, C. M., Reiss, D. J., & Hogarty, G. E. (1986). *Schizophrenia and the family.* New York: Guilford Press.

Anthony, W. A., Cohen, M. R., & Vitalo, R. (1978). The measurement of rehabilitation outcome. *Schizophrenia Bulletin, 4,* 365–383.

Bandura, A. (1969). *Principles of behavior modification.* New York: Holt, Rinehart, & Winston.

Bellack, A. S., Hersen, M., & Himmelhoch, J. M. (1983). A comparison of social skills, pharmacotherapy and psychotherapy for depression. *Behaviour Research and Therapy, 21,* 101–107.

Bellack, A. S., Hersen, M., & Lamparski, D. (1979). Roleplay tests for assessing social skills: Are they valid? Are they useful? *Journal of Counseling and Consulting Psychology, 47,* 335–342.

Bellack, A. S., Hersen, M., & Turner, S. M. (1976). Generalization effects of social skills training in chronic schizophrenia: An experimental analysis. *Behaviour Research and Therapy, 14,* 391–398.

Bellack, A. S., & Mueser, K. T. (1986). A comprehensive treatment program for schizophrenia and chronic mental illness. *Community Mental Health Journal, 22,* 175–189.

Bellack, A. S., Turner, S. M., Hersen, M., & Luber, R. F. (1984). An examination of the efficacy of social skills training for chronic schizophrenic patients. *Hospital & Community Psychiatry, 35*, 1023–1028.

Benton, M. K., & Schroeder, H. E. (1990). Social skills training with schizophrenics: A meta-analytic evaluation. *Journal of Consulting & Clinical Psychology, 58*, 741–747.

Birley, J. L. T., & Brown, G. W. (1970). Crisis and life changes preceding the onset of acute schizophrenia. *British Journal of Psychiatry, 116*, 327–333.

Blair, K., & Wallace, C. (1989). *Evaluation of the dissemination of the Medication Management Module.* (Available from Camarillo/UCLA Clinical Research Center, P. O. Box 6022, Camarillo, CA 93011–6022.)

Borland, A., McRae, J., & Lycan, C. (1989). Outcomes of five years of continuous case management. *Hospital and Community Psychiatry, 40*, 369–376.

Broen, W. E. (1968). *Schizophrenia: Research and theory.* New York: Academic Press.

Brown, G. W., Harris, T., & Peto, J. (1973). Life events and psychiatric disorders: II. Nature of the causal link. *Psychological Medicine, 3*, 159–176.

Brown, M. (1982). Maintenance and generalization issues in skills training with chronic schizophrenics. In J. P. Curran & P. M. Monti (Eds.), *Social skills training: A practical handbook for assessment and treatment* (pp. 90–116). New York: Guilford Press.

Brown, M. A., & Munford, A. M. (1983). Life skills training for chronic schizophrenics. *Journal of Nervous and Mental Disease, 17*, 1466–1476.

Cole, J. R., Klarreich, S. H., & Fryatt, M. J. (1982). Teaching interpersonal skills to adult psychiatric patients. *Cognitive Therapy and Research, 6*, 105–112.

Corrigan, P. W., MacKain, S. J., & Liberman, R. P. (In press). Skills training modules: A strategy for dissemination and utilization of a rehabilitation innovation. In J. Rothman & E. Thomas (Eds.), *Intervention research* (pp.    ). Chicago: Haworth Press.

Corrigan, P. W., Schade, M. L., & Liberman, R. P. (1991). Social skills training. In R. P. Liberman (Ed.), *Handbook of psychiatric rehabilitation.* New York: Pergamon Press.

Donahoe, C. P., Carter, M. J., Bloen, W. D., Hirsch, G. L., Laasi, N., & Wallace, C. J. (1990). Assessment of interpersonal problem-solving skills. *Psychiatry, 53*, 329–338.

Donaldson, S. R., Gelenberg, A. J., & Baldessarini, R. J. (1983). The pharmacologic treatment of schizophrenia: A progress report. *Schizophrenia Bulletin, 9*, 5–28.

Eckman, T., Liberman, R. P., Blair, K., & Phipps, C. C. (1990). Teaching medication self-management skills to chronic schizophrenics. *Journal of Clinical Psychopharmacology, 10*, 33–38.

Falloon, I. R. H. (1985). *Family management of schizophrenia*. Baltimore, MD: Johns Hopkins University Press.

Falloon, I. R. H., Boyd, J. L., McGill, C. W., et al. (1985). Family vs. individual management in the prevention of morbidity of schizophrenia. *Archives of General Psychiatry, 2*, 887–896.

Falloon, I. R. H., Boyd, J. L., McGill, C. W., Razani, J., Moss, H. B., & Gilderman, A. M. (1982). Family management in the prevention of exacerbations of schizophrenia: A controlled study. *New England Journal of Medicine, 306*, 1437–1440.

Falloon, I. R. H., & Fadden, G. (1993). *Integrated mental health care: A comprehensive community based approach*. Cambridge: Cambridge University Press.

Falloon, I. R. H., & Liberman, R. P. (1983a). Interactions between drug and psychosocial therapy in schizophrenia. *Schizophrenia Bulletin, 9*, 44–55.

Falloon, I. R. H., & Liberman, R. P. (1983b). Behavioral family interventions in the management of chronic schizophrenia. In W. R. McFarlane (Ed.), *Family therapy in schizophrenia* (pp. 223–247). New York: Guilford Press.

Falloon, I. R. H., Lindley, R., MacDonald, R., & Marks, I. M. (1977). Social skills training in outpatient groups: A controlled study of rehearsal and homework. *British Journal of Psychiatry, 131*, 599–609.

Fecteau, G. W., & Duffy, M. (1986). Social and conversational skill training with long-term psychiatric inpatients. *Psychological Reports, 59*, 1327–1331.

Fish, B. (1987). Infant predictors of the longitudinal course of schizophrenic development. *Schizophrenia Bulletin, 13*, 395–410.

Frederiksen, L. W., Jenkins, J. O., Foy, D. W., & Eisler, R. M. (1976). Social skills training to modify abusive verbal outbursts in adults. *Journal of Applied Behavior Analysis, 9*, 117–127.

Frisch, M. B., Elliott, C. H., Atsnides, J. P., et al. (1982). Social skills and stress management training to enhance patients' interpersonal competencies. *Psychotherapy: Theory, Research and Practice, 19*, 349–358.

Gjerde, P. F. (1983). Attention capacity dysfunction and arousal in schizophrenia. *Psychological Bulletin, 93*, 57–72.

Goldsmith, J. B., & McFall, R. M. (1975). Development and evaluation of an interpersonal skill-training program for psychiatric inpatients. *Journal of Abnormal Psychology, 84*, 51–58.

Gottesman, I. I., McGuffin, P., & Farmer, A. E. (1987). Clinical genetics as clues to the real genetics of schizophrenia (A decade of modest gains while playing for time). *Schizophrenia Bulletin, 13*, 23–48.

Graziano, A. M., & Katz, J. N. (1982). Training paraprofessionals. In A. S. Bellack, M. Hersen, & A. E. Kazdin (Eds.), *International handbook of behavior modification and therapy* (pp. 128–145). New York: Plenum Press.

Hansen, D. J., St. Lawrence, J. S., & Christoff, K. A. (1985). Effects of interpersonal problem-solving training with chronic aftercare patients on problem-solving component skills and effectiveness of solution. *Journal of Consulting and Clinical Psychology, 53*, 167–174.

Hersen, M., Eisler, R. M., & Miller, P. M. (1973). Development of assertive responses: Clinical measurement and research considerations. *Behavior Research and Therapy, 11*, 505–521.

Hersen, M., Eisler, R. M., & Miller, P. M. (1974). An experimental analysis of generalization in assertive training. *Behavior Research and Therapy, 12*, 295–310.

Hogarty, G. E., Anderson, C. M., & Reiss, D. J. (1987). Family psychoeducation, social skills training, and medication in schizophrenia: The long and short of it. *Psychopharmacology Bulletin, 23*, 12–13.

Hogarty, G. E., Anderson, C. M., Reiss, D. J., Kornblith, S. J., Greenwald, D. P., Javna, C. D., & Madonia, M. J. (1986). Family psychoeducation, social skills training, and maintenance chemotherapy in the aftercare treatment of schizophrenia: I. One-year effects of a controlled study on relapse and expressed emotion. *Archives of General Psychiatry, 43*, 633–642.

Holmes, M. R., Hansen, D. J., & St. Lawrence, J. S. (1984). Conversational skills training with aftercare patients in the community: Social validation and generalization. *Behavior Therapy, 15*, 84–100.

Jaffe, P. G., & Carlson, P. M. (1976). Relative efficacy of modeling and instructions in eliciting social behavior from chronic psychiatric patients. *Journal of Counseling and Clinical Psychology, 44*, 200–207.

Kazdin, A. E. (1974). Effects of covert modeling and model reinforcement on assertive behavior. *Journal of Abnormal Psychology, 83*, 240–252.

Kazdin, A. E., & Bootzin, R. R. (1972). The token economy: An evaluative review. *Journal of Applied Behavior, 5*, 343–372.

Kazdin, A. E., Matson, J. L., & Esveldt-Dawson, D. K. (1984). The relationship of role-play assessment of children's social skills to multiple measures of social competence. *Behavior Research and Therapy, 22*, 129–139.

Kindness, K., & Newton, A. (1984). Patients and social skills groups: Is social skills training enough? *Behavioral Psychotherapy, 12*, 212–222.

Klerman, G. (1977). Better but not well: Social and ethical issues in the deinstitutionalization of the mentally ill. *Schizophrenia Bulletin, 3*, 617–631.

Koh, S. (1978). Remembering in schizophrenia. In S. Schwartz (Ed.), *Language and cognition in schizophrenia* (pp. 148–162). Hillsdale, NJ: Lawrence Erlbaum.

Lamb, H. R. (1982). *Treating the long-term mentally ill*. San Francisco: Jossey-Bass.

Lehman, A. F., Ward, N. C., & Linn, L. S. (1982). Chronic mental patients: The quality of life issue. *American Journal of Psychiatry, 134*, 1271–1276.

Liberman, R. P. (1986). Coping and competence as protective factors in the vulnerability-stress model of schizophrenia. In M. J. Goldstein, I. Hand, & K. Hahlweg (Eds.), *Treatment of schizophrenia* (pp. 201–216). New York: Springer-Verlag.

Liberman, R. P. (1988). Psychiatric rehabilitation of chronic mental patients. Washington, DC: American Psychiatric Press.

Liberman, R. P. & Corrigan, P. W. (1993). *Designing new psychosocial treatments for schizophrenia. Psychiatry, 56*, 236–249.

Liberman, R. P., Corrigan, P. W., & Schade, M. L. (1989). Drug and psychosocial treatment interactions. *International Review of Psychiatry, 1*, 283–294.

Liberman, R. P., DeRisi, W., & Mueser, K. T. (1989). *Social skills training for psychiatric patients*. New York: Pergamon Press.

Liberman, R. P., Falloon, I. R. H., & Wallace, C. J. (1984). Drug-psychosocial interactions in the treatment of schizophrenia. In M. Mirabi (Ed.), *The chronically mentally ill: Research and services* (pp. 175–212). New York: Spectrum.

Liberman, R. P., King, L. W., DeRisi, W. J., & McCann, M. (1975). *Personal effectiveness*. Champaign, IL: Research Press.

Liberman, R. P., Mueser, K. T., & Wallace, C. J. (1986). Social skills training for schizophrenics at risk for relapse. *American Journal of Psychiatry, 143*, 523–526.

Liberman, R. P., Mueser, K. T., Wallace, C. J., Jacobs, H. E., Eckman, T., & Massel, H. K. (1986). Training skills in the psychiatrically disabled: Learning coping and competence. *Schizophrenia Bulletin, 12*, 631–647.

Liberman, R. P., Nuechterlein, K. H., & Wallace, C. J. (1982). Social skills training and the nature of schizophrenia. In J. P. Curran & P. M. Monti (Eds.), *Social skills training: A practical handbook for assessment and treatment*. New York: Guilford Press.

Longin, H. E., & Rooney, W. M. (1975). Teaching denial assertion to chronic hospitalized patients. *Journal of Behavior Therapy and Experimental Psychiatry, 6*, 219–222.

Lukoff, D., Snyder, K., Ventura, J., & Nuechterlein, K. (1984). Life events, familial stress, and coping in the developmental course of schizophrenia. *Schizophrenia Bulletin, 10*, 258–292.

MacKain, S. J., & Streveler, A. (1990). Social and independent living skills for psychiatric patients in a prison setting: Innovations and challenges. *Behavior Modification, 14*, 490–518.

MacKain, S. J., & Wallace, C. J. (1988). *Evaluation of social and independent living skills modules*. Los Angeles: University of California, Neuropsychiatric Institute, Clinical Research Center for Psychiatric Rehabilitation and the Study of Schizophrenia.

Marzillier, J. S., & Winter, K. (1978). Success and failure in social skills training: Individual differences. *Behavior Research and Therapy, 16*, 67–84.

McFall, R. M., & Lillesand, D. B. (1971). Behavioral rehearsal with modeling and coaching in assertion training. *Journal of Abnormal Psychology, 77*, 313–323.

McFall, R. M., & Twentyman, C. T. (1971). Four experiments on the relative contributions of rehearsal, modeling, and coaching to assertion training. *Journal of Abnormal Psychology, 81*, 199–218.

Miller, I. W., Norman, W. H., et al. (1989). Cognitive behavioral treatment of depressed inpatients. *Behavior Therapy, 20*, 25–47.

Monti, P. M., Curran, J P., Corriveau, D. P., et al., (1980). Sensitivity groups with psychiatric patients. *Journal of Consulting and Clinical Psychology, 48*, 241–248.

Morrison, R. (1990). Interpersonal dysfunction. In A. S. Bellack, M. Hersen, & A. E. Kazdin (Eds.), *International handbook of behavior modification and behavior therapy* (2nd ed.) (pp. 473–492). New York: Plenum Press.

Morrison, R. L., & Bellack, A. S (1987). The social functioning of schizophrenic patients: Clinical and research issues. *Schizophrenia Bulletin, 13*, 715–725.

Neuchterlein, K. H. (1977). Refocusing on attentional dysfunctions in schizophrenia. *Schizophrenia Bulletin, 3*, 457–469.

Neuchterlein, K. H., & Dawson, M. E. (1984). A heuristic vulnerability/stress model of schizophrenic episodes. *Schizophrenia Bulletin, 10*, 300–312.

Paul, G. L., & Lentz, R. J. (1977). *Psychosocial treatment of chronic mental patients: Milieu versus social learning programs*. Cambridge: Harvard University Press.

Randolph, E., Glynn, S. M., Eth, S., Liberman, R. P., Paz, G., Shaner, A., VanVort, W., & Escobar, J. (in press). Behavioral family management vs. customary care in the treatment of veteran schizophrenics: A clinic replication. *British Journal of Psychiatry*.

Sacuzzo, D. P. (1986). An information processing interpretation of theory and research in schizophrenia. In R. Ingram (Ed.), *Information processing approaches to clinical psychology* (pp. 98–117). New York: Academic Press.

Shepherd, G. (1986). Social skills training and schizophrenia. In C. R. Hollin & P. Trower (Eds.), *Handbook of social skills training: Clinical applications and new directions: Vol. 2* (pp. 9–38). New York: Pergamon Press.

Skinner, B. F. (1953). *Science and human behavior*. New York: MacMillan.

Spencer, P. G., Gillespie, C. R., & Ekisa, E. G. (1983). A controlled comparison of the effects of social skills training and remedial drama on the conversational skills of chronic schizophrenic inpatients. *British Journal of Psychiatry, 143*, 165–172.

Strauss, J. S., & Carpenter, W. T. (1972). The predication of outcome in schizophrenia: I. Characteristics of outcomes. *Archives of General Psychiatry, 27*, 739–746.

Strauss, J. S., & Carpenter, W. T. (1974). The prediction of outcome in schizophrenia: II. Relationships between predictor and outcome variables: A report from the World Health Organization International Pilot Study of Schizophrenia. *Archives of General Psychiatry, 31*, 37–42.

Sullivan, G., Marder, S. R., Liberman, R. P., Donahoe, C. P., & Mintz, J. (1990). Social skills and relapse history. *Psychiatry, 53*, 340–345.

Tarrier, N., & Barrowclough, C. (1990). Family interventions for schizophrenia. *Behavior Modification, 14*, 408–440.

Test, M. A. (1992). Training in community living. In R. P. Liberman (Ed.), *Handbook of psychiatric rehabilitation* (pp. 153–170). New York: Macmillan.

Torrey, E. F. (1988). Stalking the schizovirus. *Schizophrenia Bulletin, 14*, 223–230.

Vaccaro, J. V., & Liberman, R. P. (1989). Integrating skills training and case management for chronic schizophrenics in a community mental health center. In M. Bassi (Ed.), *Schizofreni e croncita* [Chronic Schiziphrenia] (pp. 13–26). Rome: CIC Edizioni Internationali.

Van Dam-Baggen, R., & Kraaimaat, F. (1986). A group social skills training program with psychiatric patients: Outcome, drop out rate, and prediction. *Behavior Research and Therapy, 34*, 161–169.

Ventura, J., Nuechterlein, K. H., & Mintz, J. (1991). A prospective study of life events in schizophrenia relapse. *Journal of Consulting & Clinical Psychology*.

Wallace, C. J. (1976). The assessment of psychotic behavior. In M. Hersen, R. Eisler, & P. Miller (Eds.), *Handbook of behavioral assessment* (pp. 315–349). New York: Academic Press.

Wallace, C. J. (1982). The social skills training program of the Mental Health Clinical Research Center for the Study of Schizophrenia. In J. P. Curran & P. M. Monti (Eds.), *Social skills training: A practical handbook for assessment and treatment* (pp. 57–89). New York: Guilford Press.

Wallace, C. J. (1988). *Adoption of innovations in mental health*. Los Angeles: University of California Clinical Research Center for the Study of Schizophrenia and Psychiatric Rehabilitation.

Wallace, C. J., Boone, S. E., Donahoe, C. P., & Foy, D. W. (1985). The chronically mentally disabled: Independent living skills training. In D. H. Barlow (Ed.), *Clinical handbook of psychological disorders* (pp. 462–501). New York: Guilford Press.

Wallace, C. J., & Liberman, R. P. (1985). Social skills training for patients with schizophrenia: A controlled clinical trial. *Psychiatry Research, 15*, 239–247.

Wallace, C. J., Liberman, R. P., MacKain, S. M., Blackwell, G., & Eckman, T. A. (1993). Modules for training social and independent living skills:

Application and impact in schizophrenia: *American Journal of Psychiatry,*
*149*, 654–658.

Weinberger, D. R., Berman, K. F., & Illowsky, B. P. (1988). Physiologic dysfunction of dorsolateral prefrontal cortex in schizophrenia: III. A new
cohort and evidence for a monoaminergic mechanism. *Archives of General Psychiatry, 45*, 609–615.

Weinberger, D. R., Berman, K. F,. & Zec, R. F. (1986). Physiologic dysfunction of dorsolateral prefrontal cortex in schizophrenia: I. Regional cerebral blood flow evidence. *Archives of General Psychiatry, 43*, 114–124.

Wirshing, W., Eckman, T., Liberman, R. P., & Marder, S. (1990) Management of risk of relapse through skills training of chronic schizophrenics.
In C. Tamminga & S. C. Schultz (Eds.), *Schizophrenia research* (pp. 255–
267). New York: Raven Press.

Zubin, J., & Spring, B. (1977). Vulnerability: A new view of schizophrenia.
*Journal of Abnormal Psychology, 86*, 103–126.

# CHAPTER 4

# Combat Stress and Post-Traumatic Stress Disorder

*Richard H. Rahe*

D ISABLING combat stress reactions have been witnessed frequently, yet codified differently, in each of our country's wars (Kellett, 1980; Mullins, 1973; U.S. Govt. Printing Office, 1870). Diagnoses for these conditions have varied from "nostalgia" in the Civil War to "shell shock" in World War I, "war neurosis" and "combat exhaustion" in World War II, and "battle fatigue" in Korea and Vietnam (Glass, 1954; Kormos, 1978). In most instances, what was described was either a precipitous or a gradual breakdown in the serviceman's ability to perform combat and other soldiering functions, accompanied by distressing and disabling body symptoms. A common assumption is that these psychological reactions, despite differing characteristics and diverse descriptive titles, comprise a single syndrome (Brill & Beebe, 1955; Grinker & Spiegel, 1945). Variability in individuals' stress parameters such as onset, symptom types, and recovery is thought to be secondary to the afflicted individual's enduring vulnerabilities, such as personality strengths and weaknesses. That is, a young, inexperienced, and frightened soldier may develop a disabling reaction during his first week in combat compared to an older, battle-knowledgeable sergeant who doesn't break down until after months of intense fighting. Treatment principles of immediacy, proximity, and expectancy are often said to apply equally in both of the above examples. Rapidly instituted, optimistic treatment provided close to the battle front, together with high expectations for return to duty, will promote recovery and good outcomes.

Drawing from the combat psychiatry literature, as well as from studies of human stress and recovery, a case can be made for distinguishing acute from chronic combat reactions (Belenky, Noy, & Solomon, 1985). In so doing, clinical presentations, precipitating factors, treatment choices, and expectations as to return to duty become more specific. Preventive mea-

83

sures for these two conditions will be seen to differ. Furthermore, it is proposed that the character and course of post-traumatic stress disorder differ for acute versus chronic psychological reactions to combat.

# ACUTE COMBAT REACTION

From their experiences in recent conflicts, the Israeli Defense Forces use the term "battle shock" to denote disabling psychological reactions to combat which appear within minutes to hours after exposure to battle. The analogue of such a reaction in a civilian setting might be "acute stress reactions" or even "panic." An *acute* combat reaction is characterized by abrupt onset; physiological hyperarousal; brief duration (minutes to hours); very high potential for life-threatening behaviors; and ready reversibility. Signs and symptoms, precipitants, treatment, and preventive measures will be presented.

## Signs and Symptoms

Signs and symptoms of acute combat reaction, from early to late in the disorder, are presented in Table 4.1. It is clear that many early manifestations of this reaction are common to all men facing battle. Therefore, it is the degree, rather than the quality, of the response that leads to a diagnosis.

One early sign is a notable reluctance of the soldier to leave a secure setting. He will be one of the last in line proceeding toward danger, casting frequent glances backwards toward safety. He may repeatedly check and recheck his equipment—such adventitial movements representing a displacement of his anxiety. The person may show a marked difficulty in understanding instructions and carrying out even simple tasks. Widely opened eyes, dilated pupils, and rapid and shallow breathing all signal an overactive sympathetic nervous system (Bachrach, 1984).

Sympathetic nervous system involvement is the major physiological component in an acute combat reaction. This is the "fight or flight" response described by W. B. Cannon (1934). If blood or urinary measures of catecholamines could be gathered from soldiers with this disorder, epinephrine and norepinephrine would be significantly and persistently elevated. Other combat stress research suggests that serum cortisol would

## TABLE 4.1  Contrast Between Acute and Chronic Combat Stress Reactions

| ACUTE COMBAT REACTION | CHRONIC COMBAT REACTION |
|---|---|
| Signs and Symptoms | |
| 1. Reluctance to leave a secure setting. | 1. Lowered frustration tolerance. |
| 2. Adventitial body movements. | 2. Excessive griping. |
| 3. Difficulty comprehending and following instructions. | 3. Loss of sense of humor. |
| 4. Sympathetic nervous system hyperarousal. | 5. Excessive alcohol and/or drug use. |
| 5. Life-threatening behaviors. | 6. Sleep disturbance, weight loss, constipation. |
| 6. Possible "overflow" of motor activity. | 7. Withdrawal from group. |
| 7. Possible seizures. | 8. Psychomotor retardation. |
| 8. Possible paralysis. | 9. 2000-yard stare. |
| 9. Overwhelming fear. | |
| Precipitants | |
| *Environmental* | |
| 1. Fatigue, hunger, cold, heat, and sleep deprivation. | 1. Fatigue, hunger, cold, heat, and sleep deprivation. |
| 2. Intensity of the battle. | 2. Duration of combat. |
| 3. Disorientation. | 3. High morbidity and mortality rates. |
| 4. Surprise. | 4. Lack of mobility/progress in battle. |
| *Interpersonal* | |
| 1. Lack of unit cohesion and esprit. | 1. Preexisting life stress. |
| 2. Lack of leadership. | 2. Loss of confidence in leadership. |
| 3. Confusion. | 3. Lack of communication. |
| 4. Reserve versus regular. | 4. Loss of group support. |
| 5. Support assignment versus front line. | |
| *Personal* | |
| 1. Age | 1. Loss of sense of purpose. |
| 2. Inexperience. | 2. Perception that no end is in sight. |
| 3. Lack of commitment to battle. | 3. Preexisting neuroses or character disorder. |
| 4. Witnessing death for first time. | |
| Treatment | |
| 1. Stop! | 1. Group support. |
| 2. Control breathing and pulse rate. | 2. Involve buddy. |
| 3. Allow victim to tell what happened once, at most twice. | 3. Attempt to modify preexisting life stresses. |

*(continued)*

**TABLE 4.1** *(continued)*

| ACUTE COMBAT REACTION | CHRONIC COMBAT REACTION |
|---|---|
| | Treatment |
| 4. Reorientation. | 5. Consider anxiolytic and hypnotic medication. |
| 5. Reestablish command structure. | |
| 6. Reestablish priorities. | 6. Consider up to 2 weeks of group therapy and physical fitness training. |
| 7. Incorporate buddy into treatment. | 7. Consider need for renewal. |
| 8. Consider rest and replenishment. | 8. Temper prognosis in accordance with preexisting psychiatric disorder. |
| 9. Expect return to duty within 48 hrs. | |
| 10. Don't place victim with physically wounded patients. | |
| | Prevention |
| | *Environmental* |
| 1. Control, where possible, fatigue, hunger, cold, and sleep loss. | 1. Control, where possible, fatigue, hunger, cold, and sleep loss. |
| 2. Prior knowledge of the battle area and conditions. | |
| | *Interpersonal* |
| 1. Group cohesion and morale. | 1. Maintenance of communication. |
| 2. Clear, easy-to-remember plans. | 2. Maintenance of morale. |
| 3. Leadership, including role models. | 3. Use of buddy system. |
| 4. Communication. | 4. Predictable periods of rest and renewal. |
| | 5. Closure after stress. |
| | *Personal* |
| 1. Realistic training. | 1. Attend to life problems before deployment. |
| 2. Mental rehearsal. | 2. Maintain physical fitness. |
| 3. Physical fitness. | 3. Pacing. |
| 4. Commitment. | 4. Conviction to cause. |
| 5. Attitude. | 5. Faith and optimism. |

also be elevated early in this reaction. Several hours into the stress situation, however, cortisol levels should revert to normal, or even low, levels (Mason et al., 1973; Mason, Sachar, & Grinker, 1965).

As the acute combat reaction worsens, the soldier may fail to take cover during an assault or remain hidden in a bunker and unable to care for a buddy in trouble. In the most severe cases, individuals may show an "overflow" of motor activity which can mimic tics and seizures. Conversely, hyperarousal can also lead to a "freezing" of motor functions, which presents as paralysis.

An acute combat reaction can develop, and resolve, in a matter of minutes. Since recovery for this condition can be extremely rapid, the soldier may show a dramatic transition from gross panic at one moment to rational thought and behavior a few minutes later. If rapid recovery fails to occur following treatment in the field, the presence of a more severe stress reaction should be suspected.

## Precipitants

It should be emphasized that no single factor can totally account for the development of an acute combat reaction. Rather, it is the sum of several forces acting in concert over a period of time. Precipitating forces may originate in the environment, they may result from interpersonal stresses, and they may emanate from the individual himself.

Environmental stresses like fatigue, hunger, cold, heat, and so forth are common experiences of soldiers. They take on additional significance when other stressful conditions also exist. For example, when intensity of battle is high and casualty rates are elevated accordingly, inordinate fear for one's life can easily surface. Add to this situation abrupt disorientation, so that the individual does not know in which direction it's safe to move, followed by a surprise enemy attack, and all of these environmental forces acting together can precipitate an acute combat reaction.

Interpersonal factors are, for the most part, a reflection of command. Seasoned combat veterans serving in close proximity to inexperienced soldiers, where they can be observed as role models, can be enormously helpful. High morale and unit cohesion have been called "the secret weapon" of the Israeli Defense Forces (Belenky, 1985). The medium which supports high morale is frequent, high-quality communication at all levels of command.

Reserve status, rather than a regular commission, and membership in a support (usually armor) rather than an elite unit, are other interpersonal precipitants of acute combat reaction. Members of elite units, where esprit and morale are generally high, tend to perform extremely well in combat (Bourne, 1970; Schifferle, 1985). Further interpersonal stress can occur when reserve soldiers are brought forward to replace the dead and injured. These reserves may be assigned to tanks which are still bloody from a recent campaign, and these soldiers find themselves communicating, by radio, with persons they've never met. In such situations, reserves have much higher rates of acute combat reaction than do regular soldiers.

Age and inexperience are also major personal precipitants of this disorder. An infantryman in his late twenties or early thirties has a much higher probability of developing an acute combat reaction than a man in his late teens or early twenties. Soldiers are especially vulnerable to acute combat reactions when they see death for the first time. Therefore, a major function of military training is to prepare soldiers for the rigors of battle so they can function, almost reflexively, in this dangerous environment. Yet it is impossible to train men for the experience of seeing their buddies killed. Finally, the length of time that men have been together is a powerful supportive force in combat and, accordingly, a predictor for low rates for acute combat reactions (Grinker & Spiegel, 1945).

A particularly difficult personal factor is assignment as a "new guy" to an already established unit. The new guy is seen as an intruder into the group and a reminder that one of their buddies has been recently killed or wounded. It may take weeks to months for the new soldier to be accepted (Glass, 1958).

## Treatment

Treatment should be immediate! It is far easier to reverse this disorder in its early stages than after the condition has become fully established. Therefore, the location where treatment is provided is frequently at, or very near, the front lines of battle. It is important to note that the person who carries out treatment is usually not a doctor. Most likely, he or she will be another soldier or a medic/corpsman.

The most important first step in treatment is to help the soldier get control over his or her hyperaroused physiology. Rapid, shallow breathing will quickly cause hypocapnia, with resultant light-headedness and further feelings of panic (Missri & Alexander, 1978). Hypothermia, hyperthermia, and tachycardia can produce similar effects. The first rule of treatment is to get the soldier to stop his motor activity—running around, talking, and blaming himself and others. Once the person begins—often literally—to "cool down," rational thinking returns quickly. Counting slowly to ten, making respiratory expirations last longer than inspirations, are both good treatment tactics. When rational thinking returns, reorientation can take place and priorities become reestablished.

An acutely stressed individual often shows a need to talk about his recent experiences. A buddy or medic should hear the story, but only once or twice. Further repetitions will have little further anxiety-reducing effects and may inadvertently reinforce the stress reaction. The soldier should then be evaluated for return to his unit (with a buddy) as opposed to rest and replenishment over the next 24 to 48 hours. These men should be treated at either a battle aid station or in a separate section of a field hospital. Medications are generally not required. Because of this condition's ready reversibility, return to duty rates can be as high as 95%.

It is a cardinal rule not to mix soldiers suffering acute psychological reactions to combat with those who are physically wounded. Men with combat stress reactions quickly identify with their wounded comrades and their psychological disabilities increase greatly. A special effort must be made to keep these two classes of patients apart; otherwise, in the normal flow of patients toward the rear, they will be cast together.

## Prevention

Environmental, interpersonal, and personal aspects of prevention should be considered, in much the same fashion as in the precipitation of this disorder. It takes effort to appreciably reduce the risk of acute combat reaction.

It is military doctrine to keep soldiers properly fed, warm, and rested whenever possible. When these conditions cannot be met, as is frequently the case in battle, the chances for acute stress reaction are slightly increased. Although resupplies may not be under the commander's control, communication with his men regarding the progress of the campaign, and the motivations and armament of the enemy are certainly under his influence. In addition, future battle plans should be phrased in language that is clear, concise, and easy to remember. Such communications will reduce the risk of acute combat reaction.

The most effective preventive force is realistic training (West, 1958). Seldom, however, is such training carried out. Perhaps the best examples of realistic training are the survival, evasion, resistance, and escape (SERE) courses conducted by the Navy and Air Force. These 1- to 2-week courses are designed for aviators, who by the nature of their duties are at high risk for capture and prisoner-of-war status. Such training has proved to be literally lifesaving for captured aviators.

Realistic training for combat soldiers could be accomplished. An important element in such training would be to allow soldiers to actually experience panic under controlled conditions. One example would be a mock poisonous gas attack. Confederates of the instructors would, on cue, run around wildly shouting "Gas!" They would then fall to the ground simulating asphyxiation. Symptoms of panic would be experienced by many in the group. Treatment of stopping and controlling physiology (allowing the return of rational thinking and action) could also be taught in a realistic setting. Mental rehearsal prior to stress training—for example, the steps a soldier should follow in a panic situation—could also be part of this training.

Physical fitness of an endurance nature results in increased parasympathetic tone (Cantor, Zillman, & Day, 1978; Keller & Seraganian, 1984). A fall in resting pulse rate and a lowering of blood pressure have been seen repeatedly in studies of persons achieving even moderate levels of endurance fitness (Cooper, 1970; Pollock, Wilmore, & Fox, 1978). Thus, enhanced parasympathetic tone secondary to physical fitness appears to act as a "brake" on sympathetic nervous system hyperarousal during panic-producing situations.

Personal commitment to battle, and a positive attitude under stress, are greatly shaped by the soldier's training. Ideally, he incorporates many of the ideals and attitudes of his instructors. It was John Wooden, the eminently successful basketball coach at UCLA, who encouraged his players to: "Be quick, but don't hurry." Such a positive attitude imparts a perception of personal control over fast-moving events, such as taking cover and returning fire while under attack.

## CHRONIC COMBAT REACTION

Conditions found in civilian life that are similar to this military entity are "chronic stress' and "burnout." The military term "combat fatigue" was, in fact, ordered into use by General Omar N. Bradley in 1943. Colonel Long writes: "Of the possible diagnostic terms discussed, this word [exhausting] was chosen because it was thought to convey the least implication of neuropsychiatric disturbance" (Mullins, 1973).

As in acute combat reaction, causes of this condition are several. Men developing chronic combat reactions have typically lived under trying conditions for weeks, months, or even years. Their psychological state appears to be characterized by hypoarousal, rather than by fight/flight. The chronic condition is typified by "conservation/withdrawal"; that is, the affected soldier frequently isolates himself from his peers and may show signs and symptoms of depression (Brill & Beebe, 1955). The "defeat situation" seen in animal models appears to be similar to combat fatigue (Henry & Stephens, 1977).

Once established, the chronic reaction is extremely difficult to reverse. Signs and symptoms, precipitants, treatment, and prevention of this disorder are presented below.

## Signs and Symptoms

Signs and symptoms of chronic combat reaction vary from early to late manifestations. Early signs include impairment of previously displayed skills, severely lowered frustration tolerance, excessive griping, and mild to moderate paranoia. As these characteristics can be frequently manifested in combat troops, it is a subtle distinction to determine when they exceed the normal range and signal concern. In a word: when these traits cause a man to significantly isolate himself from his peers, it is probably time to evaluate. Also, if there is evidence of excessive alcohol or drug use and/or signs and symptoms of depression, the diagnosis should be suspected strongly.

If urine and blood samples were collected in the field, catecholamines would likely be at normal, or even low, levels in men with chronic combat reactions. In contrast, cortisol would likely be found at significant and persistent elevations throughout the circadian cycle. In a variety of chronic stress reactions, the baseline for cortisol secretion appears to be "reset" to higher levels (Rahe, Rubin, Arthur, & Clark, 1968; Sachar, 1980). A further biochemical correlate of chronic stress is serum cholesterol. This high density lipid is frequently low during acute stress situations and high in chronic stress periods of weeks to months (Dimsdale & Herd, 1983; Rahe, Rubin, & Arthur, 1974).

A soldier stricken with chronic combat reaction in its most severe form is so slowed in his thinking and motor movements that he can be called zombie-like (Grinker & Spiegel, 1945). His vacant-eyed look, seeming to focus on a point far in the distance, has been labeled the "2000 yard stare." At this point the soldier is totally unable to function.

## Precipitants

Duration of battle as opposed to intensity, is a major precipitant in a chronic combat reaction. As in the acute disorder, high casualty rates add to the likelihood of a chronic reaction. Frequently, a direct relationship has been seen between wounded in-action rates and chronic psychological reactions to combat. One very influential environmental precipitant is lack of mobility and/or progress of the battle. This condition was widely prevalent during World War I, when trench warfare resulted in men spending as long as 2 to 3 years in the same labyrinth of tunnels. British author Robert Graves described his years in the trenches in vivid detail in *Goodbye to All That*. A few yards would be gained one day, then lost; the only quick way out of the battle was to be wounded or killed.

Interpersonal forces for this disorder include preexisting life stresses (Belenky, Tyner, & Sodetz, 1983; Belenky et al., 1985). Home and personal problems may follow the man to the front. Another interpersonal precipitant is loss of confidence in command. If a mistake in tactics is made, for example, a bombing strike hitting friendly forces, the soldier may feel that his lack of confidence is well justified. On a personal level, when a soldier loses his sense of purpose, and especially when he perceives that there is "no end in sight" to his long-lasting endeavors, the risk for this condition increases markedly. Finally, preexisting neurosis or character pathology is an additional personal factor which increases the liability of a soldier to develop a chronic combat reaction. A summary and comparison of the acute reaction with the features of chronic combat stress is depicted in Table 4.1.

## Treatment

The first approach to the treatment of this disorder is buddy and group support (Kormos, 1978). This will be most effective in the early stages of the disorder. Even then, because the affected individual is so mistrustful, it takes a strong commitment of the group to try to bring him back into the fold. Such group support has been seen to function extremely well in prisoner-of-war settings (Hubbell, 1976; Schwinn & Diehl, 1973). Here, if buddy and group efforts failed to halt the withdrawal of a fellow prisoner, that person often died. The cause of death appeared to be largely influenced by loss of hope and giving up (Kushner, 1973; Wolf & Ripley, 1974).

When specialized care is required for this condition, it means more time (a few days to 3 to 4 weeks); more professionals (psychiatrists, psychologists, and possibly exercise therapists); and more resources (medications, and a site for prolonged and specialized care) than is the case for acute combat reactions. The treatment site should be located near the front lines of battle and secure enough that it does not have to be moved frequently. The Israeli Defense Forces experimented with such a camp just inside their northern border during their Lebanon incursion. Here the men received medications (chiefly hypnotics and anxiolytics), rest and replenishment, daily group therapy, and daily group exercise sessions. This "walk 'em and talk 'em" approach resulted in return to duty rates between 40% and 70% (Belenky et al., 1985).

Therapy may also include attempts to modify pre-battle life stresses. For example, if the individual is worried about the health of his family members, some communication (preferably by telephone) should be allowed. However, personal visits, especially periods of home leave, are often counterproductive. Once the person re-enters his family setting, his resolve to return to the front lines of battle weakens and a successful resumption of duty becomes unlikely. In the long term, treatment of chronic combat reaction frequently includes a "need for renewal." Job redefinition and/or retraining is often appropriate. In animal studies of chronic stress, the defeated animal has been found to be particularly motivated to learn new behaviors (Henry & Stephens, 1977).

## Prevention

Most line commanders are cognizant of the detrimental effects of fatigue, heat, cold, hunger, and sleep deprivation on their men. Many commanders, however, are unaware of the importance of communication in a situation of long and deadly conflict. Maintenance of communication was a tremendously important support mechanism for American prisoners of war in Vietnam. By means of the chain of command, each man was given a role to carry out daily in his ongoing struggle to survive with dignity.

Another important preventive measure is establishment of predictable rest intervals. This may not be possible in some long-term battle situations; but when it is, the effects are extremely salutary. Many soldiers in Vietnam were greatly assisted in getting through their combat tours by the knowledge that they would be headed home one year to the day of their arrival. (It should be noted, however, that this policy also had undesirable effects, in that it inhibited group identity with resultant erosion of social support.)

An interpersonal preventive measure, but one frequently underemployed, is allowance for closure after a period of prolonged difficulty. Closure was done well in the days of troop ship transport home, when soldiers returned from Europe and Asia following World War II (Segal, 1973). Aboard ship, men had ample opportunities to discuss their war experiences, compare their reactions with others, and to "talk out" distressing thoughts and emotions. In a related manner, sending men to and from combat as a unit promotes both social support and closure.

In terms of personal preventive measures, one most disturbing early stress reported by prisoners of war was an awareness of things they had "left undone" prior to being taken captive (Rahe, 1987). A soldier has enough to think about during the early stages of a long-term battle without adding to his concerns over a lack of a legal will, insufficient insurance, or family problems.

Almost all persons experiencing chronic stress find physical fitness of an endurance type to be of tremendous help (Rahe & Geneder, 1983). Exercises not only help to pass time during lull periods but also maintain feelings of vigor and well-being. Of nearly equal importance is the fact that exercise greatly facilitates sleep. Finally, fitness may well counter the tendency toward hypoactivity seen in chronic combat reactions.

Perhaps the single most important personal preventive strategy for long-term stress is the development of a sense of pace. Prisoners of war and hostages held in captivity for a year or more testify to the critical importance of "taking one day at a time." Much like a mountain climber who slowly proceeds up the slope, a soldier must learn to pace himself so that sustained function is possible over many days, months, and perhaps even years. Also, like the mountain climber, he should hold some energy in reserve. Occasionally, he must draw upon these reserve energies in order to meet unexpected demands. Personal traits of acceptance, humility, and humor are also extremely important in preventing a chronic combat reaction.

A further word should be said about the incredible importance of humor in prolonged stress situations. The ability to laugh, not only with others, but at oneself, is vital. Former prisoners of war have claimed that single instances of a humorous episode would be called into their memory months later, when they most needed a good laugh (Hubell, 1976; Stockdale & Stockdale, 1984). Personal beliefs, such as conviction of cause, faith, and basic optimism, are also sustaining. Even if these characteristics are not present in individuals at the beginning of a prolonged period of stress, they frequently developed through group interactions.

## POST-TRAUMATIC STRESS DISORDER

A great deal has been written over the past decade regarding post-traumatic stress disorder (Figley, 1980; Foy, Sipprelle, & Rueger, 1984; Friedman, 1981; Sierles, Chen, McFarland, & Taylor, 1983; Walker & Cavender, 1982). As in the case of psychological reactions to combat, there appears to be an assumption that this diagnosis is a unitary one. However, from the literature on psychological reactions not only to combat, but also to disasters, it appears that there are two types of post-traumatic reactions: one secondary to acute stress and another following chronic stress.

## Acute Stress

Acute stress leading to a post-traumatic reaction is typically discrete, highly intense, and a life-threatening experience that lasts anywhere from a few minutes to a few hours. Examples include sinkings of ships, an aircraft crash, earthquakes, floods, and other natural disasters (McCaughey, 1985; Taylor & Frazer, 1982; Wilkinson, 1983). Precipitants such as confusion, disorientation, lack of communication, age, inexperience, and surprise also apply. Treatment reportedly works best if it is immediate and performed at or near the site of combat. "Return to duty" is generally encouraged to occur as soon as possible.

Post-traumatic reactions following acute stress are frequently characterized by adrenergic hyperarousal. Within a few days to weeks after the stress, victims may report hyperalertness, anxieties, startle reactions, difficulty falling asleep, and intrusive thoughts—all of which suggest high levels of circulating catecholamines (Silber, Perry, & Bloch, 1958).

Post-traumatic symptoms related to acute stress may well be part of the process of normal recovery. That is to say, recurrent disturbing thoughts and emotions secondary to the acute stress may be part of a gradual desensitization and effective processing of the stress. Patients who go on to present at a psychiatric treatment center likely represent those at the high end of a spectrum of symptomatic persons. Most individuals probably recover from an acute stress with transient and mild to moderate symptoms. Thus, the true incidence of this disorder is probably largely underestimated, while the average severity is likely overestimated.

## Chronic Stress

Post-traumatic reactions following chronic stress appear to be accompanied by signs and symptoms of depression. Affected individuals frequently complain of loss of energy, difficulties concentrating, trouble staying asleep, nightmares, poor marital and job adjustment, feelings of worthlessness, and alcoholism (Foy et al., 1984; McCaughey, 1986; Silber et al., 1958; Taylor & Frazer, 1982). This is a clinical picture of conservation/withdrawal. Moreover, the likelihood of preexisting life problems and personality liabilities of affected individuals can be part of this disorder (Figley, 1980; Sierles et al., 1983).

Chronic stress post-traumatic reaction is engendered by multiple stresses lasting over a period of months to years. Examples include prolonged combat experiences, prisoner-of-war status, and long-term hostage situations. Patients with post-traumatic reactions to chronic stress typically do not come to medical attention until months to years later (Figley, 1980; Friedman, 1981). This is not to say that these individuals do not suffer severe symptoms during the interval between cessation of the stress and arrival at a clinic. What has often precipitated the arrival for professional help is a "snowballing" of life problems. For example, Vietnam veterans with this disorder often do not approach outreach clinics until they have tried, usually unsuccessfully, for several years to adjust to civilian life. Over the years between return from the war and appearance at a clinic they have usually lost several jobs, had their marriages fall apart, gotten into financial difficulties, and perhaps found themselves on the way to alcoholism (Figley, 1980; Friedman, 1981; Sierles, 1983).

It is of interest to speculate that the hypercortisolism seen in severe depression may also be present in chronic post-traumatic stress victims. Few studies of the psychophysiology of these individuals have been carried out. Follow-up studies of prisoners of war in World War II and Korea showed that these returnees developed coronary heart disease at a significantly higher rate than did controls (Beebe, 1975). It is possible, therefore, that a prolonged elevation of serum cholesterol in response to chronic post-traumatic stress may have contributed to this accelerated development of coronary heart disease.

Some individuals' responses to stress may fall between acute and chronic reactions; these persons will show features of both disorders. For example, U.S. Navy enlisted men involved in a collision of ships at sea were seen in a psychiatric outpatient clinic some months after the accident (McCaughey, 1986). These sailors apparently had not fully recovered from the acute stress and had gone on to develop signs and symptoms of depression. Treatment objectives in these cases were first, brief attention paid to the acute stress to assess the sailors for unreasonable self-blame and guilt. Then, a shift in attention was made to address long-term issues of professional and personal readjustment (McCaughey, 1987).

The role of the psychiatrist in the prevention of post-traumatic stress disorder is a challenging one. For sufferers of acute stresses, such as victims of a disaster, the concept of rapid intervention appears to be ideal (McCaughey, 1987). The clinical focus for these victims is short-term therapy, with triage distinguishing persons with extreme reactions and/or poor coping from the majority of men and women who will recover with mild to moderate symptoms. Intervention should provide general education and mobilization of community support. Victims who are most severely disturbed should be treated intensively. Prompt treatment might well prevent, or at least moderate, post-traumatic stress disorder in this highly susceptible group. In addition, all victims should be thoroughly evaluated, both medically and psychologically (McCaughey, 1986; McCaughey, 1987; Rahe & Geneder, 1983).

For victims of chronic stress the psychiatrist's approach would be different. Following provision of immediate physical and psychological care, efforts should be directed toward facilitating closure. Group therapy and general group meetings are extremely helpful to accomplish this objective (Rahe, 1987; Rahe & Geneder, 1983). The entire group should be monitored, with yearly medical follow-up visits, over the following 5 to 10 years. The goal in treating victims of chronic stress is to find and then moderate a possible snowballing of readjustment difficulties. Work, home, and interpersonal problems are the focal issues of treatment (Segal, 1973; Solomon, Oppenheimer, & Noy, 1986; Stockdale & Stockdale, 1984; Wolf & Ripley, 1974).

## REFERENCES

Bachrach, A. J. (1984). Stress physiology and behavior under water. In C. H. Shilling, C. B. Carlson, & R. A. Mathias (Eds.), *The physician's guide to diving medicine*. New York: Plenum Press.

Beebe, G. W. (1975). Follow-up studies of World War II and Korean War prisoners. *American Journal of Epidemiology, 101*, 400–422.

Belenky, G. L., Noy, S., & Solomon, Z. (1985). Battle stress: The Israeli experience. *Military Review, 29–37*.

Belenky, G. L., Tyner, C. F., & Sodetz, F. J. (1983). *Israeli battle shock casualties: 1973 and 1982* (Report NP–83–4). Washington, DC: Walter Reed Army Institute of Research.

Bourne, P. G. (1970). *Men, stress and Vietnam*. Boston: Little, Brown.

Brill, N. Q., & Beebe, G. W. (1955). *A follow-up study of war neuroses*. Washington, DC: VA Medical Monograph.

Cannon, W. B. (1934). *Bodily changes in pain, hunger, fear, and rage*. New York: Appleton Century.

Cantor, J. R., Zillman, D., & Day, K. D. (1978). Relationship between cardiovascular fitness and physiological response to films. *Perceptual and Motor Skills, 46,* 1123–1139.

Cohen, B. M., & Cooper, M. Z. (1954). *A follow-up study of world War II prisoners of war.* Washington, DC: VA Medical Monograph.

Cooper, K. (1970). *The new aerobics.* New York: Bantam Books.

Dimsdale, J. E., & Herd, A. (1983). Variability of plasma lipids in response to emotional arousal. *Psychosomatic Medicine, 44,* 413–430.

Figley, C. A. (1980). *Strangers at home: The war, the nation, and the Vietnam veteran.* New York: Praeger.

Foy, D. W., Sipprelle, R. C., Rueger, D. B., & Carroll, E. M. (1984). Etiology of post traumatic stress disorder in Vietnam veterans: Analysis of military and combat exposure influences. *Journal of Consulting Clinical Psychology, 52,* 79–87.

Friedman, M. J. (1981). Post-Vietnam syndrome: Recognition and management. *Psychosomatics, 2,* 931–943.

Glass, A. J. (1954). Psychotherapy in the combat zone. *American Journal of Psychiatry, 110,* 725–731.

Glass, A. J. (1958). Observations upon the epidemiology of mental illness in troops during warfare. Washington, DC: U.S. Government Printing Office.

Grinker, A. A., & Spiegel, J. P. (1945). *Men under stress.* Philadelphia: Blakiston.

Henry, J. P., & Stephens, P. (1977). *Stress, health, and the social environment: A socio-biologic approach to medicine.* New York: Springer-Verlag.

Hubbell, J. G. (1976). *Prisoner of war.* New York: Reader's Digest Press.

Keller, S., & Seraganian, P. (1984). Physical fitness and autonomic reactivity to psychosocial stress. *Journal of Psychosomatic Responses, 28,* 279–287.

Kellett, A. (1980). *Combat motivation: Operational Research and Analysis Establishment* (Report No. R–77) Ottawa, Ontario, Canada: Department of National Defense.

Kentsmith, D. K. (1986). Principles of battlefield psychiatry. *Military Medicine, 151,* 89–96.

Kormos, H. R. (1978). The nature of combat stress. In C. R. Figley (Ed.), *Stress disorders among Vietnam veterans: Theory, research and treatment.* New York: Brunner/Mazel.

Kushner, F. H. (1973, April). Doctor's report from a V.C. prison. *Medical World News.*

McCaughey, B. G. (1985). U.S. Coast Guard collision at sea. *Journal of Human Stress, 111,* 43–46.

McCaughey, B. G. (1986). The psychological symptomatology of a US Naval Disaster. *Military Medicine, 151,* 162–165.

McCaughey, B. G. (1987). US Navy Special Psychiatric Rapid Intervention Team (SPRINT). *Military Medicine, 152,* 133–135.

Mason, J. W., Hartley, L. H., Kotchen, E. H., Mougey, E. H., Ricketts, P.

T., Jones L. G., Belenky, G. L., Noy, S., & Solomon, Z. (1973). Plasma cortisol and norepinephrine responses in anticipation of muscular exercise. *Psychosomatic Medicine, 35*, 406–414.

Mason, J. W., Sachar, E. J., & Grinker, A. A. (1965). Corticosteroid responses to hospital admission. *Archives of Psychiatry, 13*, 1–8.

Missri, J. C., & Alexander, S. (1978). Hyperventilation syndrome: A brief review. *JAMA, 240*, 2093–2096.

Mullins, W. S. (1973). *Neuropsychiatry in World War II: Vol. II*. Washington, DC: Office of the Surgeon General of the Army.

Nelson, P. D., & Rahe, R. H. (1987). Coping with captivity. *Proceedings of Conference on Follow-Up Care for Returning Prisoners of War* (March 12–14, 1985), San Diego, CA. Washington, DC: U.S. Government Printing Office.

Pollock, M., Wilmore, J., & Fox, S. M. (1978). *Health and fitness through physical activity*. New York: Wiley.

Rahe, R. H., & Geneder, E. (1983). Adaptation to and recovery from captivity stress. *Military Medicine, 148*, 577–585.

Rahe, R. H., Rubin, R. T., & Arthur, R. J. (1974). The three investigator study: Serum uric acid, cholesterol, and cortisol variability during the stresses of everyday life. *Psychosomatic Medicine, 36*, 358–368.

Rahe, R. H., Rubin, R. T., Arthur, R. J., & Clark, B. R. (1968). Underwater demolition team training: Serum uric acid and cholesterol variability. *JAMA, 206*, 2875–2880.

Sachar, E. J. (1980). Hormonal changes in stress and mental illness. In D. T. Krieger & J. D. Hughes (Eds.), *Neuroendocrinology*. Sunderland, MA: Sinquer Associates.

Schifferle, P. J. (1975, Nov.-Dec.). The technology of teamwork. *Armor Magazine*, 10–13.

Schwinn, M., & Diehl, B. (1973). *We came to help*. New York: Harcourt, Brace, Jovanovich.

Segal, J. (1973). Therapeutic considerations in planning the return of American POW's to the continental United States. *Military Medicine, 138*, 73–77.

Silber, E., Perry, S. E., & Bloch, D. A. (1958). Patterns of parent-child interaction in a disaster. *Psychiatry, 21*, 159–167.

Sierles, F. S., Chen, J. J., McFarland, R. E., & Taylor, M. A. (1983). Post-traumatic stress disorder and concurrent psychiatric illness: A preliminary report. *American Journal of Psychiatry, 140*, 1177–1179.

Solomon, Z., Oppenheimer, B., & Noy, S. (1986). Subsequent military adjustment of combat stress reaction casualties: A nine-year follow-up study. *Military Medicine, 151*, 8–11.

Stockdale, J., & Stockdale, S. (1984). *In love and war*. New York: Harper & Row.

Stofsel, W. (1980). Psychological sequelae in hostages and the aftercare. *Danish Medical Bulletin, 27,* 239–241.

Taylor, A. W. J., & Frazer, A. G. (1982). The stress of post-disaster body handling and victim identification work. *Journal of Human Stress, 8,* 4–12.

U.S. Government Printing Office. (1870). *Medical and surgical history of the War of the Rebellion*: Vol. I. Washington, DC.

Walker, J. L., & Cavender, J. O. (1982). Vietnam veterans: Their problems continue. *Journal of Nervous and Mental Diseases, 170,* 174–180.

West, L. J. (1958). Psychiatric aspects of training for honorable survival as a prisoner of war. *American Journal of Psychiatry, 115,* 329–336.

Wilkinson, C. B. (1983). Aftermath of a disaster: The collapse of the Hyatt Regency Hotel skywalks. *American Journal of Psychiatry, 140,* 1134–1139.

Wolf, S., & Ripley, H. S. (1974). Reactions among allied prisoners of war subjected to three years of imprisonment and torture by the Japanese. *American Journal of Psychiatry, 104,* 180–193.

# CHAPTER 5

## Psychosocial Consequences of Stress Among Native American Adolescents

*Donald W. Bechtold, Spero M. Manson, and James H. Shore*

IT is clear that many if not most Indian/Native children and adolescents live in environments and under circumstances involving significant stress. Many of these youth experience mental health problems derived at least in part from this stress and which often persists into adulthood. Yet we also know that many Indian/Native youth grow developmentally and thrive psychologically despite these stressful environments and circumstances. Such diversity of outcome, given similar and apparently comparable stressors, suggests that the variable of stress alone is not an adequate predictor of outcome. Rather, a model which considers the consequences of stress on a developing individual must account for the dynamic interplay between environmental and constitutional forces in that individual, and must recognize that some of these forces promote health while others promote pathology. In this model, the outcome of health or pathology is understood to be the result of a complex interaction between environmental forces (both stressors and protective factors) and individual forces (e.g., temperament and genetic predisposition).

In this chapter, a variety of stressors which confront Indian/Native youth are discussed. Examples include environmental stressors such as poverty, academic failure, inadequate health care, child abuse and neglect, substance abuse, teen pregnancy, and family disruption. Constitutional vulnerability, such as developmental disabilities and underlying predispositions toward affective, anxiety, and substance abuse disorders are further considered. The relationship of these underlying stressors to the development of pathology is discussed relative to such clinical conditions as suicidality, delinquency, truancy and school dropout, and runaway behaviors, as well as to specific, diagnosable DSM–III–R conditions. Finally, protective forces in the form of prevention/intervention technologies may mitigate against the pathogenic effects of both environmental stressors and psychobiologic vulnerabilities.

Public concern for the mental health of American Indian and Alaska Native youth first arose surrounding their education. *The Problem of Indian Administration*, more commonly known as the Meriam Report (Meriam, 1928), highlighted a series of school-related issues concerning the physical and emotional well-being of Indian/Native youth. Recommendations from the report included enhancement of basic standard of living, formal education surrounding Indian/Native culture, improvements in both the number and quality of school personnel, and the construction of local day schools and community centers. It was hoped that reduction of stressful daily life circumstances and improvements in educational environment would render education more relevant to Indian/Native youth. As "personal security" (self-esteem) increased, so also, the authors presumed, would academic performance.

Concerns regarding the stresses on Indian/native youth tended to abate with time following the Meriam Report and did not return with vigor until the issuance of the Kennedy Report in 1969 (U.S. Senate, 1969). At that time, the Senate Special Subcommittee on Indian Education cited a "dismal record of absenteeism, dropouts, negative self-image, low achievement, and, ultimately, academic failure" (p. 21) in considering the status of Indian/Native youth. Its recommendations were generally consistent with those of the Meriam Report, authored 40 years previously.

In subsequent years the effect of stress on Indian/Native youth began to be considered outside the educational domain. Kane and Kane (1969) advocated that the Indian Health Service (IHS) address the social and psychological welfare of Indian/Native youth with as much vigor as the infectious diseases of this population. The consequences of psychosocial stresses were thought to include alienation, adjustment difficulties, child abuse and neglect, substance abuse, and suicide. Attneave and Beiser (1974) concluded that services to children tend to be sporadically dispersed throughout IHS Mental Health programs, suggesting again that the stresses in the lives of Indian/Native youth indicated specialized mental health programming.

Concern regarding the stresses on Indian/Native youth peaked in the late 1970s. In 1976, the Children's Bureau of the Office of Human Development published a study entitled *Indian Child Welfare: A State of the Field Study*. This study, together with a volume published by the Indian Family Defense Fund (Byler, 1977), documented the rapid escalation in the placement of Indian/Native youth for custodial care with non-Indian families. The stress of disruption of the development of the child's social and cultural identity was believed to contribute to major mental health problems. The *Final Report* of the American Indian Policy Review Committee was delivered to Congress in 1977 and acknowledged that the quality of life in Indian/Native communities ranked lowest in the country by most standards. The Committee concluded that the stress of socioeconomic deprivation was a significant contributor to social disintegration, mental illness, and alcoholism. The Report of the Special Populations Subpanel on the Mental Health of American Indians and Alaska Natives (1978) reaffirmed earlier findings and added that handicapped youth, youth in the criminal justice system, and youth undergoing rapid sociocultural change experienced special mental health needs based on these additional stresses. The *Phoenix IHS Area Review: Perceptions of Service for Special Needs Children* (1986) served to remind that the effects of stress were not limited to Indian/Native adolescents but extend to younger children as well, and that services to the young lag even behind those available to youth.

Of late, national interest has turned toward the role of stress in the development of substance abuse problems in Indian/Native youth. P.L. 99–570, the Omnibus Anti-Drug Abuse Act of 1986, appropriated approximately $21.7 million to tribes to address substance abuse problems. Significant portions of these funds were earmarked for prevention as well as treatment activities, including primary and secondary preventive interventions targeted toward youth who had not yet manifested substance abuse symptomatology. Furthermore, the Omnibus Bill specifically mandated the evaluation of data pertaining to the relationship between such stresses as child abuse/neglect and substance abuse. Most recently, the Department of Health and Human Services and the Department of Labor have united in a program known as Youth 2000. The intent of this program is to increase public awareness of the stresses that imperil the healthy development of young people, to enhance their self-esteem, and to engage all sectors of the public in addressing these matters. More than 300 Indian/Native youth representing 53 tribes from 21 states met in May, 1987 under the auspices of the United National Indian Tribal Youth (UNITY) as part of this national campaign. They identified their ten most pressing concerns in order of priority: 1) substance abuse; 2) suicide; 3) teen pregnancy; 4) preservation of traditional tribal culture; 5) communication with tribal government; 6) funding for higher education; 7) motivation and self-esteem; 8) school dropout rates; 9) lack of recreational activities; and 10) unemployment. Finally, a recent survey of the Indian Education Act, Title IV, Part A programs identified the most common personal concerns prompting students to seek counseling services. In descending order of frequency, these were family problems, decision making, social conflicts, peer relationships, depression, financial difficulties, drug problems, cultural identity problems, alcohol problems, and sexual problems (Development Associates, 1983). Clearly these concerns represent either active stresses in the lives of Indian/Native youth or of outcomes to which these stresses contribute, at least in part.

Three recent studies by the National Center for American Indian and Alaska Native Mental Health Research (NCAIANMHR) add additional data (Ackerson, Dick, Manson, & Baron, 1990; Manson, Beals, Dick, & Duclos, 1989; Manson, Ackerson, Dick, Baron, & Fleming, 1990). Students at a tribally operated boarding school and a BIA boarding school and a cohort of Indian/Native students from five universities were surveyed regarding stressful life events. In general, these studies indicate that Indian/Native youth commonly experience stress both in the home and school environment. The most stressful events reported by these Indian/Native high school and college students included: 1) lack of money; 2) concern about the health of a close family member; 3) death of a family member; 4) career decisionmaking; 5) fear of failure; 6) depression; 7) concern about the personal problems of family members; 8) fear of having something stolen; 9) lack of adequate recreational activities; 10) pressure to succeed academically; 11) difficulty in dealing with intimate relationships; 12) peer pressures; and 13) pressures of acculturation. In short, it appears that Indian youth perceive stress at home, at school, in intimate relationships, in casual relationships, in relationships with authority figures, and in almost every other circumstance and environment.

It is clear that Indian/Native youth perceive stress to be fairly ubiquitous within their lives. As alluded to above, it is often difficult to separate the stressor itself from the effect of the stress on the developing youth. Such is the case in consideration of the mental health needs of Indian/Native youth: there is often close concordance in the nature, degree, and duration of stress and the subsequent development of psychopathology. At times the pathologic condition may be both resultant from previous stress and a stress in and of itself, in terms of the life functioning of the youth (e.g., dropping out of school, child abuse/neglect, delinquency, suicidal behavior, and running away from home).

There can be little doubt that stress contributes to the development of psychopathology in the terms of the *Diagnostic and Statistical Manual of the American Psychiatric Association* (3rd ed., rev.) (1987). A sizable portion of the DSM–III–R focuses on disorders first evident in infancy, childhood, and adolescence. Using a biopsychosocial model, it is understood that the relative contribution of the biologic, psychologic, and social varies from one disorder to the next. Particularly with those disorders with strong contributions from the psychosocial domain, it would be expected that with regard to prevalence rates, Indian youth are represented at least as frequently as the adolescent population at large. In actual practice, these conditions may be both underrecognized and underdiagnosed due to deficiencies in the service delivery system to Indian/Native youth; there is certainly little doubt that diagnosable psychopathology is one outcome of the stresses facing Indian/Native youth today.

Examples of conditions that would be expected to occur at relatively high rates among Indian/Native youth include:

mental retardation, which is common among socioeconomically deprived populations;

post-traumatic stress disorder, which is common among youth who have been subject to repeated abuse, neglect, and violence in their environment;

separation anxiety disorder, which is common in children who have been sensitized to loss, rejection, or abandonment;

oppositional/defiant disorder and conduct disorder, which may be seen in youth who have been consistently undersupervised in their environment;

adjustment disorders, which represent dysfunctional responses to stressful life events;

and identity disorders, in which the normal developmental process of identity formation and consolidation becomes protracted and complicated, resulting in significant distress on the part of the individual.

Identity disorder provides a useful example of the complication of normal development by the stress of the conflicting pressures of traditional versus dominant culture on the Indian/Native youth. Other conditions, such as the anxiety disorders, affective disorders, and thought disorders involve stronger biologic contributions. Solely on the basis of biologic/physiologic endowment, one would expect Indian/Native youth to manifest these conditions in rates comparable to the population at large. Furthermore, Indian/Native youth would be expected to be at significant risk and perhaps increased risk, for the development of these conditions, insofar as psychosocial stressors are known to potentiate the expression of the underlying biologic condition.

These predictions are largely borne out by the presently available data. Joe (1980) identified and evaluated 350 disabled Navajos living on or near the reservation. Three hundred two of these individuals were pre-school- or school-age youth. Their disabilities included mental retarda-tion, learning disabilities, emotional disabilities, sensory disabilities, and multiple handicaps. As a result of these and other similar data, the Native American Rehabilitation and Training Center in Flagstaff, Arizona, con-cluded that neurosensory disorders and certain developmental disabilities occur from 4 to 13 times more frequently for American Indians than for the United States population in general (1979). O'Connell (1987) used data from the 1984 study by the Office of Civil Rights and 1986 enroll-ment figures from the Bureau of Indian Affairs (BIA) to study the preva-lence of handicapping conditions among American Indian Youth. Her data reported that, for the nation as a whole, American Indians have the highest prevalence of learning disabilities, the second highest prevalence of mental retardation, and that Indian/Native students exceed the na-tional percentages in speech impairment and multiple handicaps as well.

The data likewise support the high incidence of affective illness, namely depression, among Indian/Native youth. Beiser and Attneave (1982) studied the problems of Indian youth seen through the IHS Mental Health branch as outpatients in 1974. Depression was the most common specific diagnosis among teenage girls (3rd in frequency after "not identi-fied" and "other"). May (1983) in his survey of IHS Mental Health and Social Service data from the Albuquerque area from 1979 to 1982 found that depression was diagnosed in 2.5% and 3.2% of all young people be-tween the ages of 10 and 19 seen as outpatients in 1981 and 1982 respec-tively. Furthermore, given the service delivery problems to this under-served population, it is likely that the true incidence of depression is underrepresented in these data. Kursh, Bjork, Sindell, and Nelle (1966) administered the Minnesota Multiphasic Personality Inventory (MMPI) and California Psychological Inventory (CPI) to Indian students at the Flandreau High School, a BIA Boarding School. Their findings indicated high levels of psychopathology, most commonly depression, among the students. Three recent, unpublished studies by the National Center for American Indian and Alaska Native Mental Research involved adminis-tration of a 20-item scale developed by the Center for Epidemiologic Studies (CES–D) (Radloff, 1977) to identify depressive symptoms experi-enced by student populations in a tribally operated boarding school, a BIA-operated boarding school, and a cohort including Indian/Native stu-dents from five major universities. A CES–D total score of 16 or above suggests high risk for major depression. The average CES–D score for all students in the tribally operated boarding school was 19.28, the BIA op-erated boarding school 19.53, and the University cohort 17.75. Clearly, the data suggest that depression represents both a source of stress and a response to stress on the part of a significant number of Indian/Native youth.

The data further support a high incidence of anxiety-related conditions among Indian/Native youth. Beiser and Attneave (1982) reported that anxiety occurred with almost equal frequency to depression among the youth studied. May (1983) identified anxiety in 13% and 11.3% of all youth between the ages of 10 and 19 seen as outpatients in 1981 and 1982 respectively through the Albuquerque area mental health programs of IHS. The previously referenced studies of boarding school and college students conducted by the National Center for American Indian and Alaska Native Mental Health Research demonstrated three separate dimensions of anxiety among Indian/Native youth: 1) physiologic anxiety reactions, 2) phobic reactions, and 3) performance anxiety reactions. Once again, anxiety reactions are seen both as a source of stress and a response to stress on the part of Indian/Native youth.

Numerous studies indicate that Indian/Native youth have higher use and abuse rates for nearly all types of drugs (including alcohol) than do non-Indian youth (Beauvais & Laboueff, 1985; Beauvais, Oetting, & Edwards, 1985a, 1985b; Oetting, Beauvais, & Edwards, 1988; Oetting & Goldstein, 1979). Differences in usage rates are particularly pronounced for marijuana, inhalants, and alcohol (Beauvais, Oetting, & Edwards, 1985). Oetting and Goldstein (1979) documented inhalant use by Indians as almost twice the national average in the 12- to 17-year-old group; inhalant use decreased in this study as other substances such as marijuana and alcohol became more available. Oetting and Goldstein (1979) further demonstrated that American Indian youth began abusing various substances at a younger age than did their non-Indian counterparts. Recent data show that alcohol consumption and problem drinking is extending to progressively younger children (Oetting et al., 1988; Young, 1988). Weibel-Orlando (1984) has further documented the trend toward younger age of onset as well as more rapid rates of escalation to problematic substance abuse among Indian/Native youth. Finally, a trend toward polysubstance abuse among Indian/Native youth has been shown (Oetting & Beauvais, 1985). As with the previously mentioned conditions, the bidirectional relationship between stress and substance abuse in Indian/Native youth is strongly supported.

While there is wide variation in the rate of child abuse and neglect across American Indian and Alaska Native communities, there is no doubt that this is a major source of stress among many Indian/Native youth and that this is but one in a series of significant life stressors for many youth in Indian and Native communities. Family histories of inter-personal conflict, marital disruption, parental substance abuse, parent/child attachment problems, parental unemployment, and violent death are commonly found in the background of many abused and neglected Indian children (Fischler, 1985; Ishisaka, 1978; Oakland & Kane, 1973; White & Cornely, 1981; Wischlacz, Kane, & Kempe, 1978). Indian/Native youth face additional risk of child abuse and neglect based on socio-cultural shifts such as transition away from traditional values, perceived changes in gender roles, and a changing nature of the extended family (Beiser, 1974; Graburn, 1987, Hauswald, 1987). The most extensive data to date on child abuse and neglect among Indian youth derives from a survey conducted by the Albuquerque area IHS Mental Health Programs Office and the Indian Children's Program (Piasecki, Manson, Biernoff, Hiat, Taylor, & Bechtold, 1989). The survey compared psychiatric symp-tomatology among children considered as "neglect only," "abuse only," "abuse/neglect combined," and "neither abused nor neglected," based on records and history. The abuse/neglect combined subgroup exhibited the highest psychiatric symptomatology for all symptom clusters studied. Youth in this category were found to have significantly higher incidence of depressive disorders, sleep disorders, anxiety disorders, conduct disor-ders, drug use disorders, schizotypal disorders, and developmental disor-ders. Children falling into this subgroup also demonstrated the highest frequency of expulsion from school and running away from home behav-iors. Cognitive deficits have been shown to occur more frequently in abused than nonabused children (Egeland, Sroufe, & Erickson, 1983; Martin, Beezley, Conway, & Kempe, 1974; Toro, 1982). Monane, Leich-ter, & Lewis (1984) demonstrated a higher incidence of violent behavior among abused and neglected children. Carmen, Rieker, and Mills (1984) showed an increased tendency toward self-destructive behavior on the part of abused females. It is clear that the life circumstances identified as risk factors for child abuse and neglect occur commonly in Indian/Native communities. The data furthermore strongly suggest that these life stresses coupled with abuse and/or neglect may be expressed in the form of significant psychiatric symptomatology among many Indian/Native youth.

Consideration of the psychosocial effects of stress on Indian and Native youth must include a discussion of the growing problem of suicide. The average suicide rate for American Indians and Alaska Natives from 1980 to 1982 was 19.4 per 100,000 which is 1.7 times the national average. Suicide rates for Indian/Native youth ages 10 to 14, 15 to 19, and 20 to 24 are even higher when compared to national averages: 2.8, 2.4 and 2.3

times greater, respectively (May, 1987). The highest incidence of suicide among Indian/Native people occurs among the young, as opposed to the elderly (McIntosh & Santos, 1981). There is a strong male preponderance to Indian/Native suicide as well as an association with substance abuse, highly lethal means, and an absence of strongly traditional values (Shore, 1974). A variety of significant life stresses have been shown to be risk factors for suicide among Indian/Native youth. Interpersonal conflict (Biernoff, 1969; May, 1973; Maynard & Twiss, 1970; Miller & Schoenfield, 1971; Ross & Davis, 1986), unresolved grief (Devereux, 1961; Jilek-Aall, Jilek, & Flynn, 1978), familial instability (Dizmang, Watson, May, & Bopp, 1974; May & Dizmang, 1974; Resnick & Dizmang, 1971; Swanson, Bratrude, & Brown, 1971), depression (National Task Force on Suicide in Canada, 1987; Termansen & Peters, 1979), substance abuse (Westermeyer & Brantner, 1972), and unemployment (Spaulding, 1985; Travis, 1983, 1984; Trott, Barnes, & Denoff, 1981) have been shown to increase suicide potential among Indian/Native youth. In addition, those stresses associated with a family history of psychiatric disorder, particularly alcoholism, depression, and suicide have been shown to increase youth suicide potential (Shore, Bopp, Waller, & Dawes, 1972). Multiple home placements (Berlin, 1986; Dizmang, Watson, May, & Bopp, 1974), and social disintegration, acculturation pressures, and transcultural conflicts (Hochkirchen & Jilek, 1985; Kraus & Buffler, 1979; Levy & Kunitz, 1971) may also contribute to suicidal behavior on the part of Indian/Native youth. The etiologic pathways to suicide are many. Stressful life events and circumstances are strongly represented among these pathways.

Though not in and of themselves psychiatric syndromes, school dropout, delinquency, and runaway behaviors are clearly areas of concern among Indian/Native youth. Most would agree that underlying stress, feelings of alienation, and deficient self-esteem contribute to these conditions; furthermore, these place the individual at risk for the development of more serious psychopathology. The available literature reveals that Indian/Native youth drop out from school at rates 2 to 3 times those of the general population (Developmental Associates, 1983; Grant, 1975; U.S. Department of Interior, 1976). Szasz (1974) argued that insensitivity to traditional cultural values and ideals has led Indian/Native people to perceive school as irrelevant. Hanks (1973) cited home stressors, such as the need to care for younger siblings and older family members, as contributing to this problem. Kleinfeld (1973) suggested that the high rate of parental unemployment failed to support the perception of school as vocationally necessary on the part of Indian/Native youth.

Delinquency has likewise been seen as a growing problem among Indian/Native youth. Forslund and Cranston (1975) demonstrated a high rate of delinquency characterized by a preponderance of petty offenses and misdemeanors among Indian/Native youth. May (1983) found that delinquency is more common among males than females. In addition, the runaway problem appears strongly related to delinquency among Indian/Native youth. The Indian Center, Inc. of Lincoln, Nebraska and the Department of Sociology at the University of Nebraska (1986) surveyed a cohort of runaway Indian youth and their parents. The modal runaway was found to have a history of school dysfunction, socioeconomic distress, and an absence of a strongly traditional family background. Conflict with parents and home-related problems were the predominate causes given for running away. Other causes included problems with siblings, the law, substance abuse, and peer pressures. Runaway youth commonly supported themselves through illegal means such as theft and prostitution and had extensive arrest records. Once again, the relationship with stress is unavoidable.

Clearly many Indian/Native youth function daily under enormous stressors. Often these stressors are intergenerational, having also afflicted their parents and even grandparents. Many youth respond to these stressors with dysfunctional behaviors either indicative of actual psychiatric disorder or as a risk factor for the subsequent development of psychiatric disorder. Yet, we know that many Indian/Native youth grow and thrive psychologically in spite of these adverse circumstances. The relative interplay between life stresses, biologic predisposition, and temperamental vulnerabilities remains to be fully understood. Current prevention/intervention technology has shown increasing promise for ameliorating many of the stresses described previously which affect children in general as well as Indian/Native youth. Under a contract with the Indian Health Service, 850 providers and agencies were surveyed (Manson et al., 1989) regarding the nature of ongoing preventive activities. This survey identified 194 programs actively involved in prevention activities as of May 9, 1988. Approximately one fourth of these programs are school-based, the remainder operating mainly in other human service and community settings. Tribal or Native sponsorship is present in about one half of the programs. Services range from counseling and psychotherapy to suicide prevention, substance abuse intervention, education and training, and recreational and cultural activities. Most often, these programs are aimed at mental health promotion, recognition of risk factors, reduction of stress/alleviation of situations at risk, and promotion of cultural identity. The number of programs currently active offers hope; however, outcome data are not yet available in terms of the effectiveness of these programs.

Beiser and Manson (1987) reviewed and evaluated the primary prevention programs aimed at emotional and behavioral disorders in Native children. They classified programs according to their area of focus, namely, family, school and community. With regard to family interventions, they described an exemplary child abuse and neglect demonstration project implemented by the Northern Cheyenne which demonstrated substantial increases in reporting and self-referrals, a reduction in foster home placements, improved interagency coordination, and community support. Regarding school-based interventions, Beiser and Manson described a recreational therapy program designed to reduce student risk for depression, substance abuse, truancy, and antisocial behavior based at the Chemawa Indian Boarding School in the Pacific Northwest. So successful was this program, which included activities such as hot air ballooning, kayaking, and climbing, that it was extended, first to include activities during the summer break, and ultimately incorporated into the orientation process for new students.

Teen health centers are described as a popular example of community-based intervention in Native communities. Beiser and Manson (1989) offer the Acoma-Canoncito-Laguna Teen Center as one successful example. This center offers services such as health education, counseling, a library, exercise classes, acne and weight control programs, special workshops for teens and their parents, and in-service training for professionals involved in service delivery to the teens of the community. Though longer-term and more carefully controlled outcome studies are clearly indicated, Beiser and Manson's review engenders optimism that appropriately selected and applied preventive interventions will impact favorably in attempts to mitigate against the effects of stress so ubiquitous in the lives of Native children and adolescents. Consequently, there are data which suggest that well-reasoned and carefully planned applications of this technology may serve to alleviate, at least in part, the oppressive effect of these stresses on Indian/Native youth.

# ACKNOWLEDGMENTS

The preparation of this manuscript was supported in part by NIMH MH19156–03, NIMH MH42473–07, and NIMH MH00833–03.

# REFERENCES

Ackerson, L. M., Dick, R. W., Manson, S. M., & Baron, A. E. (1990). Depression among American Indian adolescents: Psychometric characteristics of the Inventory to Diagnose Depression. *Journal of the American Academy of Child and Adolescent Psychiatry, 29,* 601–607.

American Psychiatric Association. (1987). *Diagnostic and statistical manual of mental disorders* (3rd ed. rev.) Washington, DC: Author.

Attneave, C. L., & Beiser, M. (1974). *Service networks and patterns of utilization, mental health programs, Indian Health Service.* (Unpublished report submitted to the Indian Health Service).

Beauvais, F., & Laboueff, S. (1985). Drug and alcohol abuse intervention in American Indian communities. *The International Journal of the Addictions, 20,* 139–171.

Beauvais, F., Oetting, E. R., & Edwards, R. W. (1985a). Trends in drug use of Indian adolescents living on reservations: 1975–1983. *American Journal of Drug and Alcohol Abuse, 11,* 209–229.

Beauvais, F., Oetting, E. R., & Edwards, R. W. (1985b). Trends in the use of inhalants among American Indian adolescents. *White Cloud Journal, 3,* 3–11.

Beiser, M. (1974). Hazard to mental health: Indian boarding schools. *American Journal of Psychiatry, 131,* 305–306.

Beiser, M., & Attneave, C. L. (1982). Mental disorders among Native American children: Rate and risk periods for entering treatment. *American Journal of Psychiatry, 139,* 193–198.

Beiser, M., & Manson, S. M. (1987). Prevention of emotional and behavioral disorders in North American Native children. *Journal of Preventive Psychiatry, 3,* 225–240.

Berlin, I. N. (1986). Psychopathology and its antecedents among America Indian adolescents. *Advances in Clinical Child Psychology, 9,* 125–152.

Biernoff, M. (1969). *A report on Pueblo Indian suicide.* Unpublished manuscript.

Byler, W. (1977). The destruction of American Indian families. In S. Unger (Ed.), *The destruction of the American Indian Family* (pp. 1–11). New York: The Association on American Indian Affairs.

Carmen, E., Rieker, P., & Mills, T. (1984). Victims of violence and psychiatric illness. *American Journal of Psychiatry, 141,* 378–383.

Development Associates (1983). *Final report: The evaluation of the impact of the Part A entitlement program funded under Title IV of the Indian Education Act.* Arlington, VA: Author.

Devereux, G. (1961). *Mohave ethnopsychiatry.* Washington, DC: Smithsonian Institution Press.

Dizmang, L. H., Watson, J., May, P. A., & Bopp, J. (1974). Suicide in the American Indian. *Psychiatric Annals, 4,* 22–28.

Egeland, B., Sroufe, L. A., & Erickson, M. (1983). The developmental consequence of different patterns of maltreatment. *Child Abuse & Neglect, 7*, 459–469.

Fischler, R. (1985). Child abuse and neglect in American Indian communities. *Child Abuse & Neglect, 9*, 95–106.

Forslund, M. A., & Cranston, V. A. (1975). A self-report comparison of Indian and Anglo delinquency in Wyoming. *Criminology, 13*, 193–197.

Graburn, N. (1987). Severe child abuse among the Canadian Inuit. In N. Scheper-Hughes (Ed.), *Child Survival* (pp. 211–225). Norwell, MA: Kluwer Academic Publications.

Grant, W. V. (1975). Estimates of school dropouts. *American Education, 11*, 42.

Hanks, G. A. (1973). Dependency among Alaska Native school dropouts. In B. E. Oviatt, (Ed.), *A perspective of the Alaskan Native school dropout*. Salt Lake City: Social Service Resource Center of Utah. (ERIC Document Reproduction Service No. ED 116876.)

Hauswald, L. (1987). External pressure/internal change: Child neglect on the Navajo reservation. In M. Scheper-Hughes (Ed.), *Child Survival* (pp. 145–164). Norwell, MA: Kluwer Academic Publications.

Hochkirchen, B., & Jilek, W. (1985). Psychosocial dimensions of suicide and parasuicide in American Indians of the Pacific Northwest. *Journal of Operational Psychiatry, 16*, 24–28.

Indian Center, Inc. (Lincoln, NE), & Bureau of Sociological Research, University of Nebraska (Lincoln). (1986, July). The Native American adolescent health project: Report on interview surveys of runaways, parents, community leaders and human service workers. Unpublished report.

Ishisaka, H. (1978). American Indians in foster care: Cultural factors and separation. *Child Welfare, 57*, 299–308.

Jilek-Aall, L., Jilek, W. G., & Flynn, F. (1978). Sex role, culture, and psychotherapy: A comparative study of three ethnic groups in Western Canada. *Journal of Psychological Anthropology, 4*, 473–488.

Joe, J. R. (1980). *Disabled children in Navajo society*. Ann Arbor, MI: University Microfilms International.

Kane, R. L., & Kane, R. A. (1972). *Federal health care (with reservations!)*. New York: Springer Publishing.

Kleinfeld, J. (1973). *A long way from home: Effects of public high schools on village children away from home*. Fairbanks, AK: Institute of Social, Economic, and Government Research. (ERIC Document Reproduction Service No. ED 087581.)

Kraus, R., & Buffler, P. (1979). Sociocultural stress and the American Native in Alaska: An analysis of the changing patterns of psychiatric illness and alcohol abuse among Alaska Natives. *Culture, Medicine and Psychiatry, 3*, 111–151.

Kursh, T. P., Bjork, J., Sindell, P. S., & Nelle, J. (1966). Some thoughts on the formation of personality disorder: Study of an Indian boarding school. *American Journal of Psychiatry, 122*, 868–876.

Levy, J., & Kunitz, S. (1971). Indian reservations, anomie, and social pathologies. *Southwestern Journal of Anthropology, 27*, 97–128.

Manson, S. M., Ackerson, L. M., Dick, R., Baron, A. E., & Fleming, C. M. (1990). Depressive symptoms among American Indian adolescents: Psychometric characteristics of the Center for Epidemiologic Studies Depression Scale (CES–D). *Psychological Assessment, 2*, 231–237.

Manson, S. M., Beals, J., Dick, R. W., & Duclos, C. W. (1989). Risk factors for suicide among Indian adolescents at a boarding school. *Public Health Reports, 104*, 609–614.

Martin, H., Beezley, P., Conway, E., & Kempe, H. (1974). The development of abused children. *Advances in Pediatrics, 21*, 25–73.

May, P. A. (1983). *A survey of the existing data on mental health in Albuquerque Area*. Unpublished report.

May, P. A. (1987). Suicide and self-destruction among American Indian youths. *American Indian and Alaska Native Mental Health Research, 1*, 52–69.

May, P. A. (1973). *Suicide and suicide attempts on the Pine Ridge Reservation*. Pine Ridge, SD: P.H.S. Community Mental Health Program.

May, P. A., & Dizmang, L. H. (1974). Suicide and the American Indian. *Psychiatric Annals, 4*, 22–28.

Maynard, E., & Twiss, G. (1970). Suicide attempts. In *That these people may live: Conditions Among the Oglala Sioux of the Pine Ridge Reservation* (DHEW Publication No. HSM 72–508). Washington, DC: U.S. Government Printing Office.

McIntosh, J. L., & Santos, J. F. (1981). Suicide among minority elderly: A preliminary investigation. *Suicide and Life Threatening Behavior, 11*, 151–166.

Meriam, L. (1928). *The problem of Indian administration*. Baltimore, MD: Johns Hopkins Press.

Miller, S. I., & Schoenfeld, L. (1971). Suicide attempt patterns among the Navajo Indians. *International Journal of Social Psychiatry, 17*, 189–193.

Monane, M., Leichter, D., & Lewis, D. (1984). Physical abuse in psychiatrically hospitalized children and adolescents. *This Journal, 23*, 653–658.

National Task Force on Suicide in Canada (1987). *Suicide in Canada*. Ottawa, Ontario, Canada: Health and Welfare Canada.

*Native American Rehabilitation and Training Center*. (1979). Unpublished program report.

Oakland, L., & Kane, R. (1973). The working mother and child: Neglect on the Navajo Reservation. *Pediatrics, 51*, 849–853.

O'Connell, J. C. (Ed.). (1987). *A study of the special problems and needs of American Indians with handicaps both on and off the reservation*. Report submitted to the U.S. Department of Education, Office of Special Education and Rehabilitative Services.

Oetting, E., & Beavais, F. (1985, September). *Epidemiology and correlates of alcohol use among Indian adolescents living on reservations*. Paper presented at the National Institute on Alcohol Abuse and Alcoholism conference (theme: Epidemiology of alcohol use and abuse among U.S. ethnic minority groups), Bethesda, MD.

Oetting, E., Beauvais, F., & Edwards, R. W. (1988). Alcohol and Indian youth: Social and psychological correlates and prevention. *Journal of Drug Issues, 18*, 87–101.

Oetting, E. R., & Goldstein, G. S. (1979). Drug use among Native American adolescents. In G. Beschner & A. Friedman (Eds.), *Youth drug abuse*. Lexington, MA: Lexington Books.

*Phoenix IHS Area Review: Perceptions of service for special needs children*. (1986). Unpublished report. U.S. Department of Health and Human Services, Indian Health Service.

Piasecki, J. M., Manson, S. M., Biernoff, M. P., Hiat, A. B., Taylor, S. S., & Bechtold, D. W. (1989). Abuse and neglect of American Indian children: Findings from a survey of federal providers. *American Indian and Alaska Native Mental Health Research, 3*, 43–62.

President's Commission on Mental Health. (1978). *The Report of the Special Populations Subpanel on the Mental Health of American Indians and Alaska Natives*. Washington, DC: U.S. Government Printing Office.

Radloff, L. S. (1977). A CES–D scale: A self-report depression scale for research in the general population. *Applied Psychological Measurement, 1*, 385–401.

Resnick, H. L., & Dizmang, L. H. (1971). Suicidal behavior among American Indians. *American Journal of Psychiatry, 127*, 882–887.

Ross, C. A., & Davis, B. (1986). Suicide and parasuicide in a Northern Canada Native community. *Canadian Journal of Psychiatry, 3*, 331–334.

Shore, J. H. (1974). Psychiatric epidemiology among American Indians. *Psychiatric Annals, 4*, 56–66.

Shore, J. H., Bopp, J. E., Waller, T. R., & Dawes, J. W. (1972). A suicide prevention center on an Indian reservation. *American Journal of Psychiatry, 128*, 1086–1091.

Spaulding, J. M. (1985). Recent suicide rates among ten Ojibwa Indian bands in Northwestern Ontario. *Omega, 16*, 347–354.

Swanson, D. W., Bratrude, A. P., & Brown, E. M. (1971). Alcoholism in a population of Indian children. *Diseases of the Nervous System, 32*, 835–842.

Szasz, M. C. (1974). *Education and the American Indian*. Albuquerque, NM: University of New Mexico Press.

Termansen, P. E., & Peters, R. W. (1979, August). *Suicide and attempted suicide among Status Indians in British Columbia*. Paper presented at the meeting of the World Federation for Mental Health congress, Salzburg, Austria.

Toro, P. (1982). Developmental effects of child abuse: A review. *Child Abuse & Neglect, 6,* 423–431.

Travis, R. (1983). Suicide in Northwest Alaska, *White Cloud Journal, 3,* 23–30.

Travis, R. (1984). Suicide and economic development among the Inupiat Eskimo. *White Cloud Journal, 3,* 14–21.

Trott, L., Barnes, G., & Denoff, R. (1981). Ethnicity and other demographic characteristics as predictors of sudden drug-related deaths. *Journal of Studies on Alcohol, 42,* 564–78.

U.S. Congress. (1977). *American Indian Policy Review Commission: Final Report.* (vol. 1). Washington, DC: U.S. Government Printing Office.

U.S. Department of Health, Education, and Welfare, Office of Human Development, Office of Child Development, Children's Bureau. (1976). *Indian child welfare: A state-of-the field study.* DHEW Pub. No. (OHD) 76–30095. Washington, DC: Government Printing Office.

U.S. Department of Interior, Bureau of Indian Affairs. (1976). *Research and Evaluation Report Series* (No. 42.00).

U.S. Senate (1969). *Indian education: A national tragedy: a national challenge.* Committee on Labor and Public Welfare, Special Subcommittee on Indian Education.

Weibel-Orlando, J. (1984). Substance abuse among American Indian youth: A continuing crisis. *Journal of Drug Issues, 14,* 313–335.

Westermeyer, J., & Brantner, J. (1972). Violent death and alcohol use among the Chippewa in Minnesota. *Minnesota Medicine, 55,* 749–752.

White, R., & Cornely, D. (1981). Navajo child abuse and neglect study: A comparison group examination of abuse and neglect of Navajo children. *Child Abuse & Neglect, 5,* 9–17.

Wischlacz, C., Lane, J., & Kempe, C. (1978). Indian child welfare: A community team approach to protective services. *Child Abuse & Neglect, 2,* 29–35.

Young, T. J. (1988). Substance use and abuse among Native Americans. *Clinical Psychology Review, 8,* 125–138.

# CHAPTER 6

# Psychiatric Implications of Stressful Methods Employed by Totalist Cults

*Louis Jolyon West*

## INTRODUCTION

UNDER influence of certain kinds of stressors or duress, individuals can be made to comply with the demands of those in power. They can also be induced to adopt beliefs and behaviors far different from those which were characteristic of them before the stress was applied. Terms like brainwashing, thought reform, coercive persuasion, and mind control have been employed to describe these processes and to account for the consequential changes in personality and behavior. In the past, such terms—and the processes they defined—referred mainly to techniques for influencing prisoners of war, political detainees, hostages held by terrorists, and the like. Recently, however, similar methods have been used by leaders of totalist cults to recruit, retain and exploit members.

Most of the people who join cults might have become more vulnerable to recruitment at a time of life change, loneliness, or disorientation. However, it is also true that cults seek out people who are considered vulnerable for precisely these reasons. Once identified, the targets are then subjected to deliberate and powerful recruitment techniques that increase their vulnerability and make them dependent upon the group. Observers who fail to recognize the stressful pressures employed by cults to recruit and retain members may focus only on the member/victim and their putative weaknesses or personality characteristics, thereby engaging in a well-known process that has been called "blaming the victim."

Persons who have been exposed to such conditions may suffer considerable harm—psychological, physical, financial, and other—as a consequence of having been thus manipulated and controlled. Their families, friends, and communities are also likely to suffer. The nature of the cult problem, the stressful techniques that cults employ to bind and exploit

117

their members, the types of psychopathology exhibited by cult victims, and approaches to their treatment are the latest observations in a series of studies which began with those prisoners of war in whom the late Ransom J. Arthur had such an important interest.

## Brainwashing

"Brainwashing" has come to mean "intensive indoctrination . . . in an attempt to induce someone to give up basic political, social or religious beliefs and attitudes and accept contrasting regimented ideas." The term is sometimes employed in a narrower sense, connoting forcible and prolonged procedures, including mental torture, or sometimes in a far broader sense, as "to persuade by propaganda" (Webster's Third New International Dictionary of the English Language, 1966, p. 267)

Numerous books and scientific papers describe the details of techniques that have come to be called variously brainwashing, thought control, mind control, political or religious conversion, etc., and the psychological and social processes involved. Among the more useful are the contributions of Hunter (1951, 1956), Hinkle and Wolff (1956), West (1957), Farber, Harlow, and West (1957), Chen (1960), Lifton (1961), Biderman and Zimmer (1961), Schein (1961), and Frank (1961). During the Korean War these techniques were used to influence Western prisoners in efforts to induce various compliant behaviors, some of which were then exploited by the captors for propaganda purposes.

The English word "brainwashing" was created by an American journalist (Hunter, 1951), from Chinese ideographs that are perhaps more usefully and less pejoratively translated as "thought reform" (Lifton, 1961). Originally, brainwashing referred to a technique for political indoctrination of small groups of people—not necessarily prisoners—in order to rid them of previously practiced "wrong thinking" and convert them to Communism, or at least make them sympathetic to Marxist beliefs. This method helped Mao Tse-tung and his followers to win over the Chinese people to their cause. Torture and deliberate mistreatment were not necessarily part of this procedure.

During and after the Korean War, however, the term "brainwashing" as used in the West became expanded to mean almost any procedure employed to induce compliant behaviors (including expressions of changed political belief, and false confessions) in prisoners or other dominated individuals. Thus both nonviolent group methods of changing political views and cruelly stressful procedures to break the will of isolated pris-

oners were lumped together and called brainwashing. Some of the implications for both society and science of this semantic elaboration are discussed elsewhere (Farber, Harlow, & West, 1957; Hinkle & Wolff, 1956;
West, 1957, 1962, 1964; West, Janszen, Lester, & Cornelison, 1962).

While perhaps justified by humane concern or political outrage, more
extravagant interpretations of brainwashing with attendant formulations
of mechanism, whether primarily physiological (Sargant, 1961) or psychological (Meerloo, 1951) have not proved very useful in the long run.
True, Meerloo's concept of "menticide" has also made it to the
dictionary:

> a systematic and intentional undermining of a person's conscious
> mind for the purpose of instilling doubt and replacing that doubt
> with ideas and attitudes directly inimical to his normal ideas and
> attitudes by subjecting him to mental and physical torture, exten-
> sive interrogation, suggestion, training and narcotics . . . (Web-
> ster, 1966, p. 1412)

Nevertheless, the contributions of Lifton (1961), of Biderman (1963),
and of Schein (1961) have better stood the test of time.

## STRESSORS RELEVANT TO UNDERSTANDING CULTS

Today, in nontechnical literature, such words as "brainwashing" and
even less flamboyant terms such as "thought reform" and "coercive persuasion" have been somewhat superseded by the more colloquial "mind
control." This term is now often employed to account for the domina-
tion and manipulation by certain cults of their members. It is hard for
people to understand how the followers of Jim Jones, L. Ron Hubbard,
Sun Myung Moon, Rajneesh and such are induced to do what they do,
without involving the idea of mind control. A recent upsurge of interest
in this general topic perhaps derives also from growing legal efforts to obtain recovery for damages by those who claim to have been controlled
and victimized by cult leaders or cultic organizations, with resultant
harm, suffering, or loss.

Some say that legal claims of this type (torts) invoking accusations of
mind control should be rejected. These critics argue that without physical
coercion nobody can be persuaded to follow an exploitive person or join
a cultic group, to participate in its activities, or to remain in it for a protracted period of time—often despite the pleas of family and friends—

against his* will or because of mind control. Further, the argument goes, it cannot be shown that such joining, participating, and remaining, in and of themselves can do any harm.

Herewith support is given to the opposite view. I argue that under certain stressors people can be deliberately manipulated, influenced, and controlled to a considerable degree, even to their detriment, and induced to express beliefs and exhibit behaviors far different from what their lives up to then would logically or reasonably have predicted possible. In addition, there is evidence that persons in such situations may indeed suffer harm—psychological, physical, financial and other—as a consequence of having been thus manipulated, influenced, and controlled. Furthermore, derivatives of such harm may be experienced by other people, especially business partners, family members, other loved ones, or even in a larger sense by the community as a whole.

## Communication and Control

For more than three millennia people have been aware that they can deliberately affect the mood, thought, and behavior of others by special environmental settings and meaningful words. During the last 50 years many experimental and naturalistic observations have expanded our appreciation of the power inherent in apperceived communications, and of the many variables which intervene between the transmission of any message and its final consequences, both within the person of the recipient and upon that recipient's behavior. The flow of information is modulated in its effectiveness by a great variety of attendant variables. These variables include, *inter alia*, the age of the recipient; his relationship to the source of communication and his attitude toward it; his level of intelligence; his emotional state; his previous experience, mental set, or sensitization with regard to the subject matter and the source; and the characteristics of the situation in which communication takes place.

## Hypnotic Suggestion and the Demand Characteristics of Situations

Nowhere in the history of science is the potential impact of communication on bodily function more dramatically demonstrated than in research

---

*The detached masculine pronoun is used throughout in the traditional convention to designate both sexes.

on hypnosis. In the 1840s, for example, a British surgeon named James Esdaile reported approximately 300 major surgical procedures and more than 1000 minor ones carried out upon patients who were magnetized or mesmerized (Braid's term "hypnosis" had not yet been introduced) without the patients' wincing or exhibiting other signs of pain such as increased pulse rate, rapid breathing, or dilation of the pupils (Esdaile, 1846). In one modern experiment (West, Niell, & Hardy, 1952), it was shown that hypnotic anesthesia is not only a progressive function of the effectiveness of verbal communication (i.e., the depth of hypnosis), but that it is also accompanied by a profound suppression of involuntary autonomic nervous system functions, such as the GSR. Furthermore, even when verbal suggestions do not result in anesthesia, or even in a change in pain threshold, galvanic skin response (GSR—an index of sympathetic nerve activity elicited by painful stimuli) may be significantly reduced. While the mechanisms of psychophysiological action in hypnosis are not fully understood, from the time of Pierre Janet and Morton Prince their connection with dissociation (see below) has been well established (Bliss, 1986; Spiegel, 1986, 1991; West, 1960, 1967).

The therapeutic power of verbal and nonverbal interpersonal suggestions, as exemplified in hypnosis and other forms of suggestive therapeutics, is to be found throughout the long history of the healing arts. However, it should also be recognized that malign suggestions can have the opposite effect, as described in the literature on voodoo death and a host of related phenomena, right down to the harmful consequences of inept communications by doctors to patients (e.g., "At the most you have three months to live.") (Barber, 1961; Cannon, 1942; Cohen, 1985; Dimsdale, 1977; Eastwell, 1987; Golden, 1977; Hall, 1986; Richter, 1957; Wintrob, 1973). It has been shown in the laboratory that hypnotic suggestion alone can produce untoward physical reactions (e.g., blisters of the skin, elevations of blood pressure, increased secretions of gastric acid, etc.) and a variety of mental and emotional aberrations as well (Deckert & West, 1963).

It is also possible through hypnotic suggestion to create distortion of values, viewpoints, or perceptions of reality, sufficient to induce, in some subjects, extraordinary behaviors—even including criminal acts—that would be otherwise unacceptable to them (Kline, 1972; Orne, 1972; Watkins, 1972). One need not limit this observation to laboratory studies. Clinical experience is replete with examples of increased suggestibility or controllability of individuals during altered states of awareness induced by psychotropic substances, environmental manipulations, and other special circumstances.

## Stressor Effects of Environmental Manipulation

In this century, the efficacy of contrived environmental settings to amplify the power of communication in affecting the behavioral state of animals was pioneered by Pavlov and subsequently by generations of experimental psychologists and physiologists. More recently such influences on the feelings, thoughts, and behaviors of individuals have been demonstrated by a number of experiments. Orne (1969) showed that it is possible to hypnotize people without their knowledge, and without giving them specific suggestions, if the subjects are influenced by the demand characteristics of the situation in such a way as to appreciate—at some level of consciousness—what is expected or required of them. Other modern medical hypnotists like Harold Rosen, Jerome Schneck, Milton Erikson, William Kroger, Lewis Wolberg, Ainslie Meares, Fred Frankel, David Spiegel, and many others have employed the suggestive therapeutics of hypnosis without classical trance induction.

Milgram (1974) showed that subjects could be induced to commit various egregious acts, such as administering apparently unbearable pain to others, under conditions where it seemed to have been authorized by someone else. Zimbardo, Haney, Banks, and Jaffe (1973) demonstrated the power both of role-playing and special settings. In this now classic experiment, a group of psychologically stable volunteer subjects was randomly assigned to play the role of either prisoner or guard. Within a week, some of the "prisoners" had become so nervous and depressed that they had to be released from the experiment; meanwhile, some of the "guards" had become so callous and brutal that it was feared they might harm somebody, and the experiment had to be aborted. There are other examples in the psychological literature (see Allen, 1965; Asch, 1952; Moscovici, 1976; Tuddenham, 1958; Zimbardo, Ebbesen, & Maslach, 1977). I know of some even more drastic examples (e.g., certain military training exercises) that have never been published.

The efficacy of social settings was even more vividly demonstrated by the brainwashing or thought reform program of the Chinese Communists. This method relied upon small group dynamics, the structure of the group, the relationship of the dominant leader to the dependent members, the relative initial isolation of each individual from other members of the group, and the evolution of a growing group identity and group pressure to bring errant members into line. O'Neill and Demos (1977) have likened the first step in the thought reform process to the creation of an identity crisis. The manipulators then undertake to establish desired cognitive habits in the subject by the use of verbal reconditioning. Subjects are forced to communicate verbally and continuously, but in a process of communication which is strictly controlled. As a result, an identity crisis is forced. In my view, a new pseudo-identity may then emerge and endure as long as the demand characteristics of the situation require it.

From observations after the Korean War of returning American POWs (and subsequently of other prisoners as well) it became clear that the relative success of techniques to elicit false confessions, self-denunciations, and participation in propaganda activities was in great part achieved because of the captors' control over the environment of the prisoners, especially to the extent that this control, mediated by contriving a variety of stresses, produced in the captives a state of dependency. The role of dependency—particularly with regard to information flow and interpersonal support—has assumed increasing importance in studies of the phenomenology of psychosocial influence in various circumstances, including those of totalist cults in the United States.

## The Stockholm Syndrome: Effect of Captivity on Civilian Hostages

Civilian hostage situations further illustrate circumstances wherein the attitudes and personalities of captives are affected by situational dynamics. Like the Korean War POWs, civilian victims are subjected to special stressors, in situations from which (at least for a time) there is no escape, wherein they become dependent upon their captors for physical and psychological needs.

Ochberg (1978) and Strentz (1980) have described one of the psychological sequelae of becoming a hostage as the Stockholm syndrome (a term which Ochberg attributes to Special Agent Conrad Hassel of the FBI) after an attempted bank robbery in Sweden. Several customers and bank employees were held captive in a Stockholm bank for several days in 1974. During the ordeal one woman hostage fell in love with one of her captors and publicly berated the Swedish prime minister for his failure to understand her captor's point of view. This hostage continued to express affection for her captor for a time after her release. Other hostages also revealed their sympathy for—or identification with—their captors.

The term "Stockholm syndrome" has since been applied to a number of hostage situations. For example, in 1975, during the 13-day seizure of a Dutch train by South Moluccan gunmen demanding freedom for their islands in the Malay archipelago, some of the captives experienced rapid development of feelings of affection or sympathy for their murderous captors, along with attitudes of distrust for their own (Dutch) authorities. Perhaps a more psychologically descriptive phrase for this phenomenon (invented for somewhat different purposes during World War II by Anna Freud) would be "identification with the aggressor."

Hard-to-explain feelings of sympathy and even identification with one's captors have been described by such former victims as Hungary's Jozseph Cardinal Mindszenty, Judge Giuseppe Digennaro (an Italian magistrate held by members of the Red Brigade), Dr. Tiede Herrema (captured by Gallagher and Coyle of the Irish Republican Army), and many others. Factors that seem to promote the Stockholm syndrome of identification with the aggressor are the intensity of the experience; its duration; the dependence of the hostage on his captor; and special characteristics of the situation, including the psychological distance of the hostage from his normal environment.

Symonds (1980) has used the phrase "frozen fright" to describe a paralysis of will in which victims feel completely trapped as they respond to sudden overwhelming danger. He describes a triad of (1) being in a hostile environment; (2) becoming isolated; and (3) feeling helpless. As a result, victims respond with regressed or childlike adaptive behavior, sometimes called traumatic infantilism. This may cause a victim to cling to the very person endangering his life. Such freezing has long been classified by psychiatrists as a dissociative reaction.

The conditions of captivity or coercive indoctrination are likely to be experienced as psychologically traumatic events, outside the range of usual experience. Post-traumatic stress disorder (PTSD) may result. The American Psychiatric Association's *Diagnostic and Statistical Manual of Mental Disorders* (3rd ed., revised) (*DSM–III–R*) states that such traumata may involve serious threats to life or physical integrity, such as natural or deliberately caused disasters (e.g., torture, death camps); a serious threat or harm to close relatives or friends; or seeing another person who has recently been, or is being, violently injured or killed. In some cases, the trauma may come from merely learning about a danger or harm to a close friend or relative. More subtle forms of trauma may be occasioned by a complete disruption of life circumstances, being cut off from usual channels of communication and orientation, being bombarded by strange or unusual stimuli, etc., as employed by contemporary totalist cults in controlling, transforming, and exploiting their members.

## Cult Indoctrination and Induction of Stress

Psychopathologists have perceived the cult type of situation to generate a form of PTSD in which dissociative features are likely to be prominent.

Dissociative disorders feature "a disturbance or alteration in the normally integrative functions of identity, memory, or consciousness" (APA, 1987, p. 277). Symptoms such as trance states, depersonalization, partial amnesia, feelings of unreality, emotional numbness, or an altered sense of identity are recognized by the DSM–III–R in "dissociated states that may occur in people who have been subjected to periods of prolonged and intensive coercive persuasion (e.g., brainwashing, thought reform, or indoctrination while the captive of terrorists or cultists)" (p. 277). Methods similar to those employed by the Chinese Communists in their thought reform programs have been used to recruit and indoctrinate members into totalist cults. Such an organization has been defined as follows:

> Cult (totalist type): a group or movement exhibiting a great or excessive devotion or dedication to some person, idea, or thing, and employing unethical, manipulative or coercive techniques of persuasion and control (e.g., isolation from former friends and family, debilitation, use of special methods to heighten suggestibility and subservience, powerful group pressures, information management, promotion of total dependency on the group and fear of leaving it, suspension of individuality and critical judgement etc.), designed to advance the goals of the group's leaders, to the possible or actual detriment of members, their families, or the community." (West, 1989)

There may be some differences in the intensity of the cult's persuasive activities, and in the degree of its effectiveness in separating a recruit from his previous social support network. Yet, successful indoctrination of a cult member is likely to include many elements similar to political indoctrination as described by Schein (1961). The following is a list of stressors known to increase the captive's—or recruit's—susceptibility, and could apply to either circumstance:

1) isolation of the subject and manipulation of his environment;
2) control over channels of communication and information;
3) debilitation through fatigue and inadequate diet;
4) degradation or diminution of the self;
5) induction of uncertainty, fear, and confusion, with joy and certainty through surrender to the group as the goal;
6) alternation of harshness and leniency in a context of discipline;
7) peer pressure, often applied through ritualized struggle sessions, generating guilt and requiring confessions;

8) insistence by seemingly all-powerful hosts that the recruit's survival—physical or spiritual—depends on identifying with the group;

9) assignment of monotonous tasks or repetitive activities, such as chanting, staring while immobilized, long chains of simple responses to simple commands, or endless copying of written materials; and

10) acts of symbolic betrayal or renunciation of self, family, and previously held values, designed to increase the psychological distance between the recruit and his previous way of life.

A report issued by the Vatican entitled *Sects or New Religious Movements* (1986) expressed the concern of Catholic scholars about the influence of totalist religious groups (i.e., cults), and names a number of elements in the process of such induced change in behavior and belief. The Vatican Report covers much of the same ground as that summarized above.

> Some recruitment, training techniques, and indoctrination procedures practiced by a number of sects and cults, which often are highly sophisticated, partly account for their success. Those most often attracted by such measures are those who, firstly, do not know that the approach is often staged, and, secondly, are unaware of the nature of the contrived conversion and training methods (the social and psychological manipulation) to which they are subjected. The sects often impose their own norms of thinking, feeling, and behaving. This is in contrast to the church's approach which implies full-capacity informed consent.

> Young and elderly alike who are at loose ends are easy prey to those techniques and methods, which are often a combination of *affection* and *deception* (cf. the *love-bombing*, the *personality test* or the *surrender*). These techniques proceed from a positive approach but gradually achieve a type of mind control through the use of abusive behavior modification techniques.

> The following elements are to be listed:

> - subtle process of introduction of the convert and his gradual discovery of the real hosts;
> - overpowering techniques: love-bombing, offering a free meal at an international center for friends, flirting-fishing technique (prostitution as a method of recruitment);
> - ready-made answers and decisions are being almost forced upon the recruits;
> - flattery;

- distribution of money, medicine;
- requirement of unconditional surrender to the initiator, leader;
- isolation: control of rational thinking process, elimination of outside information and influence (family, friends, newspapers, magazines, television, radio, medical treatment, etc.) which might break the spell of involvement and the process of absorption of feelings and attitudes and patterns of behavior;
- processing recruits away from their past lives; focusing on past deviant behavior such as drug use, sexual misdeeds; playing upon psychological hang-ups, poor social relationships, etc.;
- consciousness-altering methods leading to cognitive disturbances (intellectual bombardment); use of thought-stopping clichés, closed system of logic; restriction of reflective thinking;
- keeping the recruits constantly busy and never alone; continual exhortation and training in order to arrive at an exalted spiritual status, altered consciousness, automatic submission to directives; stifling resistance and negativity; response to fear in a way that greater fear is aroused;
- strong focus on the leader; some groups may even downgrade the role of Christ in favor of the founder (in the case of some Christian sects) (Secretariat for Promoting Christian Unity, 1986).

# VULNERABILITY TO CULT-EMPLOYED STRESSORS

## Cult Recruitment

There are several different views concerning the most important factors in the cult recruitment process, especially with regard to the roles of the leaders, the members, and the organizations in question. Some are inclined to assume that those who enter cults drift into them 1) in search for relief from symptoms of psychopathology, 2) as an escape from a bad family situation, or 3) to find an oasis of peace in a stressful and violent society. Included is the attribution of temporary situational vulnerability (e.g., the potential recruit has just moved to a new city and is without his usual interpersonal support network; he has just experienced some personal loss; he is on vacation alone; he is experiencing a difficult adjustment to college; etc.). Ungerleider and Wellisch (1979) borrowed Lifton's (1961) term, ideological hunger, to describe a common psychosocial characteristic of 50 individuals they studied who were members or former members of a variety of religious cults. However, other investigators have found that many former cult members recall no such ideological hunger as a personal characteristic prior to recruitment into the cult. Once in, it is commonly suggested to the recruit that he had such a need, but didn't realize it until his indoctrinators revealed it to him.

Some appear to believe sincerely that even the strangest of cults may be serving a helpful purpose, functioning perhaps as therapeutic communities or sheltered workshops for neurotic or schizoid youngsters, former drug abusers, or sufferers from existential anomie. Some studies report that a significant portion of those who become involved in cults were maladjusted, troubled, or even psychiatrically ill beforehand. For example, in a study undertaken with the cooperation of the Unification Church, Deutsch and Miller (1983) examined four female members and found all of them to have certain qualities—difficulties with heterosexual relations, idealism and the wish to serve or unify with others, a spiritual world view, and a tendency to deny negative or threatening stimuli—which, the investigators suggested, had attracted them to the life style and doctrines of the "sect." Levine (1981) concluded from a series of studies that alienation, demoralization, and low self-esteem made some individuals particularly vulnerable to groups that offered salvation and answers to life's problems. In my view, such studies suffer from the same flaw as that which may invalidate the conclusions of Ungerleider and Wellisch (1979)—at least with respect to a great many of those indoctrinated by cults.

Many commentators such as those referenced above view the cult not as an active agent, but rather as a passive entity which just happens to be there and is sought out by the recruit. When one attributes various characteristics to those who are drawn into cults, without looking at the forceful maneuvers employed by the cults to recruit and retain members, one may be "blaming the victim." If an offense is explained primarily in terms of characteristics of the victim, the behavior of the perpetrator need not be analyzed.

Let me reiterate that cultic studies which rely on current members' reports of life before joining must be inspected with great caution. People often feel the need to reconcile their past history, beliefs, and attitudes with present behavior to diminish cognitive dissonance. Furthermore, most if not all totalist cults require their members to reject the outside world, and especially their former lives, including family and friends, attitudes and values, as evil, unhealthy, or inadequate. Therefore, cult members may tell horror stories about their pre-cult lives that are replete with retrospective distortions, outright lies, and omissions of everything positive, all to meet the cult's specifications for what life outside must be, and thus what their pre-cult life must have been.

Many observers, including the author, believe that in fact most of the adolescents and young adults who join cults were not seriously disturbed to begin with. They might have become more vulnerable to recruitment at a time of life change, loneliness, or disorientation (after a move to a new city, or university, or simply while traveling); but it is also true that cults seek out people who are considered vulnerable for precisely these reasons, and therefore cast their nets in these waters. Once identified, the target will be subjected to powerful recruitment techniques.

Many reports fail to consider the deliberate practices of totalist cults, and the power of their methods to recruit, retain, and control normal, ordinary young people. One might even employ the term "enslave;" because this type of exploitation and control has no closer analogy in contemporary society. During the recruiting process in some cults people are encouraged to criticize themselves in small group confessionals as a means of strengthening their dependence. As the process continues, members are systematically trained to relinquish independent action and thought. Obedient behaviors and passive attitudes are rewarded. Even groups which may originate as therapeutic communities, such as Synanon, can evolve into totalist cults if the autonomy of the members is progressively diminished while the concentration of power in the leadership grows and grows.

## Psychiatric Sequelae

Reports of harmful influence exercised by cults upon their members have been supported by journalistic investigations, by law enforcement agencies, and by legislative inquiries. In addition, there are numerous published accounts by mental health professionals of symptoms observed in the course of therapy of individuals who left cults voluntarily or were "deprogramed" (Clark, 1978; Etemad, 1979; Galper, 1981; Goldberg & Goldberg, 1982; Langone, 1983; Singer, 1978).

Certainly the psychiatric symptoms seen in people emerging from totalist cults often meet the criteria for post-traumatic stress disorder. Dissociative features are usually prominent, with additional signs including disturbance or alteration in the normally integrative functions of identity, memory, or consciousness. Such a disturbance or alteration may be sudden or gradual, transient or chronic, immediate or delayed. Six features of the so-called cult indoctrination syndrome have been described (West & Singer, 1980) to include the following:

1. Sudden, drastic alteration of the victim's value system.
2. Reduction of cognitive flexibility and adaptability.
3. Narrowing, blunting or distortion of affect.
4. Psychological regression.
5. Physical changes, including weight loss, deterioration in physical appearance, mask-like facial expression, with a blank stare or darting, evasive eyes, or a puppet-like cheeriness.
6. In some cases, clear-cut psychopathological changes including major dissociative symptoms, obsessional ruminations, delusional thinking, hallucinations and various other psychiatric signs and symptoms. (p. 3249)

Much of the past decade's debate about cults has dealt with the conflict between concerns over harm to members and their families versus the claims of religious organizations to First Amendment protection. These issues have been discussed elsewhere by Delgado (1977), West and Delgado (1978), West (1989), and many others; they will not be reviewed here. Instead, let me explain that, as a physician, I look at the problem of brainwashing or coercive persuasion or mind control, whether or not in relation to the phenomenology of cults, with health and disease in mind. In my judgment, based on clinical experience, many people in these cultic organizations are at risk. Many are already sick. The burden upon their families generates additional psychiatric casualties. The numbers of such casualties are steadily mounting. There is physical morbidity to consider as well, and a number of deaths. Unfortunately, the health-related professions remain largely ignorant of these issues, and the question of legal remedies for victims of totalist cults is in a state of confusion.

# COPING WITH CULTS

## Medicolegal Aspects

For damage done by cults to their members and members' families, as for other harmful improprieties, there should be potent social and legal remedies, deriving both from the recent evolution of a consumer protection tradition (as exemplified in the health field) and from the older legal matrix of redress for grievances and civil wrongs. If a member or a former member of a cult finds that he has been mentally or emotionally harmed as a result of having been in the group, he should be able to sue that organization and/or its leader for the damages or losses he has experienced. To be sure, if he hopes to win a recovery for such damages or losses, he must develop proof, which can require investigations, witnesses, experts from psychiatry or related fields, and courtroom procedures. If proof is forthcoming, then such a lawsuit should lead to a recovery. Ten years ago such suits were very rare. Recently, some have been successful. If lawsuits of this type increasingly lead to recovery of damages from totalist cults, the epidemic of cult-related harms may begin to subside, as cult victims and their families are provided greater protection under the law.

The process of legal retribution, including payment of damages or reparations, has been found to be effective in the therapy of death-camp survivors, former hostages, and victims of torture and terrorism. In the United States, the Alien Tort Claims Act of 1979 (28 U.S.C. 1350) holds that victims of torture can sue their torturers. Stofsel (1980) has described his experience treating victims of the 1975 and 1977 hijackings of trains in Holland. A special aftercare program, funded by the Dutch government, was established to help victims and their families in the process of readjustment. The aftercare team found that more serious short-term effects occurred when victims simply tried to "forget" their ordeal, than when counseling was accepted. The team found also that financial compensation represented a psychologically helpful proof of vindication to these victims, many of whom had felt themselves to be "unpaid soldiers" of the state. In a recent South African case a white student leader, Auret Van Heerden, sued ten officers of the Security Police in an action for damages, claiming a post-traumatic stress disorder (PTSD) induced by torture in detention. The Afrikaaner judge ruled that the diagnosis was proved, and that PTSD had indeed resulted from the conditions of detention. This was psychologically very helpful to the victim, even though, for technical reasons, a large monetary recovery was not forthcoming. Former victims of the ousted military regime in Argentina have been observed to benefit in a similar way from legal actions against their former persecutors.

Much of the current controversy about brainwashing or mind control relates to whether it is truly possible for cultic groups or authority figures to influence and control the thoughts and behaviors of followers to their detriment. It should be added that in religious cults a special aura of doubt prevails, deriving both from the mystical content of putative religious teachings and practices and from First Amendment considerations. In the secular world, however, there is general acceptance that detrimental influence and control can be real. Intimidation through force or threat of force is a powerful dominator of behavior, and thoughts tend to follow behavior through rationalization and self-justification. Deception is also a well-known method of exploiting people through misinformation, concealment, distraction, or betrayal of trust. Our laws and codes of ethics accept the vulnerability of people to intimidation and deception. They also accept the possibility that relationships of special trust (such as those enjoyed by physicians, nurses, psychologists, other health workers, attorneys, and ministers) may be improperly exploited.

Generally the courts have required that the wronged person recognize and declare his victimization. He must produce evidence that he has been swindled, cheated, harmed, or damaged, and then seek legal redress. Maybe he wins his case; maybe he doesn't. The court might decide that he should have read the fine print, or that he didn't exercise reasonable prudence. Despite consumer protection laws, *caveat emptor* still obtains. Nevertheless, in traditional cases the reality and effectiveness of intimidation and deception are not at issue. Someone does it to the victim; he does not do it to himself. The argument presently confronting us proposes that the alleged victim of mind control by a cult such as the People's Temple (Jonestown), the Unification Church, the Hare Krishnas, the Divine Light Mission, the Church Universal and Triumphant, the Children of God, or the Church of Scientology, in some way does it to himself; the result is that the cult is blameless under the law. Only if it can be argued that the cult member is incompetent, and his family can persuade a court to appoint a conservator, is it possible legally to remove from the cult someone who has been rendered compliant by the powerful methods used to hold him in seemingly willing bondage.

## Organized Attempts to Deal with Cults

An international conference for scholars of the cult problem recently reviewed many aspects of social policy related to it (West & Langone, 1985). Among other actions the conference endorsed the resolution, shown in Table 6.1, which was adopted by the 1982 National Convention of the U.S. Parents & Teachers Association (PTA). Surprisingly few psychiatrists, even child psychiatrists, or other mental health professionals seem to be aware of this position statement by the PTA.

On May 22, 1984, the European Parliament adopted a resolution on "New Organizations Operating Under the Protection Afforded to Religious Bodies." This resolution expressed the Parliament's concern about

**TABLE 6.1 Resolution Adopted by National Congress of Parents and Teachers Association (PTA), 1982.***

CULTS

Whereas, various cults often recruit members by deceptive means; and

Whereas, cults often keep their members by using mind control and by alienating the members from their families; and

Whereas, many families have deep emotional scars caused by their childrens' dependence on cults; and

Whereas, an awareness of the recruitment and retention techniques of cults could help prevent a young person's entry into cults; therefore be it

*Resolved*

That the national PTA urge state PTA's/PTSA's and their units to hold education programs to inform families and youth about methods of recruitment, and techniques used to exercise control over members' thoughts and actions by cults; and be it further

*Resolved*

That the national PTA provide a list of available resources to assist state PTA's/PTSA's and their local units in planning such programs.

*National Congress of Parents and Teachers. (1982). Cults. Resolution adopted in 1982 by National Convention.

the recruitment and treatment of members of cultist organizations and called for an exchange of information among member states on problems arising from the activities of these groups. Particular reference was made to charity status and tax exemption; labor and social security laws; missing persons; infringement of personal freedoms; existence of legal loopholes which enable proscribed activities to be pursued from one country to another; and creation of centers to provide those who leave the organization in question with legal aid, assistance with social reintegration, and help in finding employment.

The resolution stated that "the validity of religious beliefs is not in question, but rather the lawfulness of the practices used to recruit new members and the treatment they receive." It went on to urge member states to pool their information about such organizations as a prelude to developing "ways of ensuring effective protection of Community citizens." To achieve this, the resolution recommended that the criteria listed in Table 6.2 be applied in investigating, reviewing, and assessing the activities of the above mentioned organizations. The resolution concluded by stating that it is desirable to develop "a common approach within the context of the Council of Europe," and "calls, therefore, on the governments of the Member States to press for appropriate agreements to be drawn up by the Council of Europe which will guarantee the individual effective protection from possible machinations by those organizations and their physical or mental coercion."

## CONCLUSION

Totalist cults are able to operate successfully—and profitably—because their recruits are unaware of the subtle but powerful stressors to which they are being subjected. At any given time most cult members are either not yet aware that they are being victimized or, having come to realize it, are unable to express such awareness because of fear, uncertainty, shame, or impairment of will secondary to post-traumatic stress disorder or dissociative disorder. In such cases, the impairment is itself a consequence of the deceptive practices and subsequent stressful forces involved in member recruitment and retention. It is extremely difficult for people thus damaged to initiate legal actions on their own behalf. However, on behalf of those who can and do seek legal remedies, on behalf of their families, on behalf of the multitudes still in bondage, and those not yet recruited but currently exposed to risk, the legitimacy of such legal actions should be confirmed by the American courts with the help of knowledgeable experts from the mental health-related professions. If more attorneys interested in civil rights would turn their sympathies and skills to the representation of such victims, important advances could be made. Progress in this field also depends heavily on the prospect that psychiatrists and other mental health workers will take greater interest in the psychopathology and psychotherapy of cult victims, as these patients and their families increasingly turn to the health professions to help them cope with the immediate and long-term sequelae of cult victimization.

## TABLE 6.2  Criteria for Assessing Suspected Cults*

(a) persons under the age of majority should not be forced, on becoming a member of an organization, to make a solemn, long-term commitment that will determine the course of their lives;

(b) there should be an inadequate period of reflection on financial or personal commitment involved;

(c) after joining an organization, contacts must be allowed with family and friends;

(d) members who have already commenced a course of education should not be prevented from completing it;

(e) the following rights of the individual must be respected;

  –the right to leave an organization unhindered;
  –the right to contact family and friends in person or by letter and telephone;
  –the right to seek independent advice, legal or otherwise;
  –the right to seek medical attention at any time;

(f) no one may be incited to break any law, particularly with regard to fundraising, for example by begging or prostitution;

(g) organizations may not extract personal commitments from potential recruits, for example students or tourists, who are visitors to a country which they are not a resident;

(h) during recruitment, the name and principles of the organization should always be made immediately clear;

(i) such organizations must inform the competent authorities on request of the address or whereabouts of individual members;

(j) the above-mentioned organizations must ensure that individuals dependent on them and working on their behalf receive the social security benefits provided in the Member States in which they live or work;

(k) if a member travels abroad in search of the interest of an organization, it must accept responsibility for bringing the individual home, especially in the event of illness;

(l) telephone calls and letters from members' families must be immediately passed on to them;

(m) where recruits have children, organizations must do their utmost to further their education and health, and avoid any circumstances in which the children's well-being might be at risk.

*Adopted from the May 22, 1984 Resolution of the European Parliament (1984), ''New Organizations Operating Under the Protection Afforded to Religious Bodies.''

# REFERENCES

Allen, V. L. (1965). Situational factors in conformity. In L. Berkowitz (Ed.), *Advances in experimental social psychiatry: Vol. 2* (pp. 133–175). New York: Academic Press.

American Psychiatric Association. (1987). *Diagnostic and statistical manual of mental disorders* (3rd ed., rev.). Washington, DC: Author.

Asch, S. E. (1952). *Effects of group pressure upon the modification and distortion of judgement*. New York: Holt, Rinehart, and Winston.

Barber, T. X. (1961). Death by suggestion. *Psychosomatic Medicine, 23*, 153–155.

Biderman, A. D. (1963). *March to calumny: The story of American POWs in the Korean War*. New York: Macmillan.

Biderman, A. D., & Zimmer, H. (1961). *The manipulation of human behavior*. New York: John Wiley.

Bliss, E. L. (1986). *Multiple personality, allied disorders and hypnosis*. New York: Oxford University Press.

Cannon, W. B. (1942). "Voodoo" death. *American Anthropologist, 44*, 169–177.

Chen, T. E. H. (1960). *Thought reform of the Chinese intellectuals*. New York: Oxford University Press.

Clark, J. G. (1978). Problems in referral of cult members. *Journal of the National Association of Private Psychiatric Hospitals, 9*, 27.

Cohen, S. I. (1985). Psychosomatic death: Voodoo death in a modern perspective. *Integrative Psychiatry, 3*, 46–51.

Deckert, G. H., & West, L. J. (1963). Hypnosis and experimental pathology. *American Journal of Clinical Hypnosis, 4*, 256–276.

Delgado, R. (1977). Religious totalism: Gentle and ungentle persuasion under the First Amendment. *Southern California Law Review, 51*, 1.

Deutsch, A., & Miller, M. J. (1983). A clinical study of four Unification Church members. *American Journal of Psychiatry, 140*, 767–770.

Dimsdale, J. E. (1977). Emotional causes of death. *American Journal of Psychiatry, 134*, 1361–1366.

Eastwell, H. D. (1987). Voodoo death in Australian Aborigines. *Psychiatric Medicine, 5*, 71–73.

Esdaile, J. (1846). *Mesmerism in India and its practical application in surgery and medicine*. London: Longman, Brown, Green, & Longman.

Etemad, B. (1979). Extrication from cultism. In J. Masserman (Ed.), *Current psychiatric therapies*: Vol. 18 (pp. 217–223). New York: Grune and Stratton.

European Parliament. (1984). New Organization Operating Under the Protection Afforded to Religious Bodies. Resolution, PE 90.562, adopted May 22, 1984.

Farber, I. E., Harlow, H. F., & West, L. J. (1957). Brainwashing, conditioning and DDD: Debility, dependency, and dread. *Sociometry, 20*, 271–285.

Frank, J. D. (1961). *Persuasion and health*. New York: McGraw Hill.

Galper, M. (1981). The cult phenomenon: Behavioral science perspectives applied to therapy. *Marriage and Family Review, 4*, 141–149.

Goldberg, L., & Goldberg, W. (1982). Group work with former cultists. *Journal of the National Association of Social Workers, 27*, 165–170.

Golden, K. M. (1977). Voodoo in Africa and the United States. *American Journal of Psychiatry, 134*, 1425–1427.

Hall, H. (1986). Suggestion and illness. *International Journal of Psychosomatics, 33*, 24–27.

Harlow, H. (1974). *Learning to love*. New York: Aronson.

Hinkle, I. E., & Wolff, H. G. (1956). Communist interrogation and indoctrination of enemies of the state. *AMA Archives of Neurology and Psychiatry, 76*, 115–174.

Hunter, E. (1951). *Brainwashing in Red China*. New York: Vanguard.

Hunter, E. (1956). *Brainwashing: The story of men Who defied it*. New York: Pyramid Books.

Kline, M. V. (1972). The production of antisocial behavior through hypnosis: New clinical data. *International Journal of Clinical and Experimental Hypnosis, 20*, 165–174.

Langone, M. (1983). Treatment of individuals and families touched by cult involvement. *Update, 7*, 27–38.

Levine, S. (1981). Cults and mental health: Clinical conclusions. *Canadian Journal of Psychiatry, 26*, 534–539.

Lifton, R. J. (1961). *Thought reform and the psychology of totalism*. New York: W. W. Norton.

Meerloo, J. A. M. (1951). The crime of menticide. *American Journal of Psychiatry, 107*, 594–598.

Milgram, S. (1974). *Obedience to authority: An experimental view*. New York: Harper and Row.

Moscovici, S. (1976). *Social influence and social change*. New York: Academic Press.

Ochberg, F. M. (1978). The victim of terrorism. *Practitioner, 220*, 293–302.

O'Neill, W. F., & Demos, G. D. (1977). The semantics of thought reform. *Etc. 34*, 413–430.

Orne, M. T. (1969). Demand characteristics and quasicontrols. In R. Rosenthal & R. Rosnow (Eds.), *Artifact in social research* (pp. 143–179). New York: Academic Press.

Orne, M. T. (1972). Can a hypnotized subject be compelled to carry out otherwise unacceptable behavior? *International Journal of Clinical and Experimental Hypnosis, 20*, 101–117.

Richter, C. P. (1957). On the phenomenon of sudden death in animals and man. *Psychosomatic Medicine, 19*, 191–198.

Sargant, W. (1961). *Battle for the mind*. Baltimore: Penguin.

Schein, E. H. (1961). *Coercive persuasion*. New York: W. W. Norton.

Secretariat for Promoting Christian Unity, Rome, (1986, May 3). *Sects or New Religious Movements*. (Publication No. 100). Washington, DC: United States Catholic Conference.

Singer, M. T. (1978). Therapy with ex-cult members. *Journal of the National Association of Private Psychiatric Hospitals, 9*, 13.

Spiegel, D. (1986). Dissociating damage. *American Journal of Clinical Hypnosis, 29*, 123–131.

Spiegel, D. (1991). Neurophysiological correlates of hypnosis and dissociation. *Journal of Neuropsychiatry and Clinical Neurosciences, 3*, 440–445.

Stofsel, W. (1980). Psychological sequelae in hostages and the aftercare. *Danish Medical Bulletin, 27*, 239–241.

Strentz, T. (1980). The Stockholm syndrome: Law enforcement policy and ego defenses of the hostage. *Annals of the New York Academy of Science, 347*, 137–150.

Symonds, M. (1980). Acute responses of victims to terror. *Evaluation and Change. Special Issue*, 39–41.

Tuddenham, R. D. (1958). The influence of a distorted group norm upon individual judgement. *Journal of Psychology, 46*, 227–241.

Ungerleider, J. T., & Wellisch, D. K. (1979). Coercive persuasion (brainwashing), religious cults, and deprogramming. *American Journal of Psychiatry, 163*, 279–282.

Watkins, J. G. (1972). Antisocial behavior under hypnosis: Possible or impossible? *International Journal of Clinical and Experimental Hypnosis, 20*, 95–100.

*Webster's third new international dictionary of the English language* (Unabridged). (1966). Springfield, MA: G. & C. Merriam.

West, L. J. (1957). United States Air Force prisoners of the Chinese communists. In *Methods of forceful indoctrination: Observations and interviews, Symposium No. 4*, pp. 270–284. New York: Group for the Advancement of Psychiatry.

West, L. J. (1960). Psychophysiology of hypnosis. *Journal of the American Medical Association, 172*, 672–675.

West, L. J. (1962). Some psychiatric aspects of civil defense. In G. W. Baker & L. S. Cottrell (Eds.), *Behavioral science and civil defense* (pp. 81–91). Washington, DC: National Academy of Sciences, National Research Council.

West, L. J. (1964). Psychiatry, "brainwashing," and the American character. *American Journal of Psychiatry, 120*, 842–850.

West, L. J. (1967). Dissociative reaction. In A. M. Freedman and H. I. Kaplan (Eds.), *Comprehensive textbook of psychiatry* (pp. 885–899). Baltimore: Williams and Wilkins.

West, L. J. (1989). Persuasive techniques in contemporary cults. In M. Galanter (Ed.), *Cults and new religious movements* (pp. 165–192). Washington, DC: American Psychiatric Press.

West, L. J., & Delgado, R. (1978, November 26). Psyching out for the cults' collective mania. *Los Angeles Times*.

West, L. J., Janszen, H. H., Lester, B. K., & Cornelison, F. S. (1962). The psychosis of sleep deprivation. *Annals of the New York Academy of Sciences, 96*, 66–70.

West, L. J., & Langone, M. D. (1985). *Cultism: A conference for scholars and policy makers*. Summary of proceedings of the Wingspread Conference on Cultism, September 9–11. Weston, MA: American Family Foundation.

West, L. J., Niell, K. C., and Hardy, J. D. (1952). Effects of hypnotic suggestion on pain perception and galvanic skin responses. *Archives of Neurology and Psychiatry, 68*, 549–560.

West, L. J., & Singer, M. T. (1980). Cults, quacks, and nonprofessional psychotherapies. In H. I. Kaplan, A. M. Freedman, & B. C. Sadock (Eds.), *Comprehensive textbook of psychiatry* (pp. 3245–3258). Baltimore: Williams and Wilkins.

Wintrob, R. M. (1973). The influence of others: Witchcraft and rootwork as explanations of behavior disturbances. *Journal of Nervous and Mental Disease, 156*, 318–326.

Zimbardo, P. G., Ebbesen, E. B., & Maslach, C. (1977). Influencing attitudes and changing behavior: An introduction to method, theory, and applications of social control and personal power. Reading, MA: Addison-Wesley.

Zimbardo, P. G., Haney, C., Banks, W. C., & Jaffe, D. (1973, April 8). The mind is a formidable jailer: A Pirandellian prison. *New York Times*, pp. 38–60.

# CHAPTER 7

## The Psychology of Terrorism and Torture in War and Peace: Diagnosis and Treatment of Victims

*Calvin J. Frederick*

## THE NATURE OF TERRORISM

T ERRORISM is by no means a geography-specific phenomenon and has always attracted a wide spectrum of participating activists. Ironically, its efficiency has been nurtured by modern progress in the transportation and communications industries, since it is now possible to communicate around the world in minutes or seconds. Modern technology and transportation provide virtually limitless combinations of networks for terrorists to make maximal use of present-day developments. Major airline bombings, where the perpetrators were thousands of miles away, bear tragic witness to these facts. Terrorism has become a sophisticated, omnipresent phenomenon. In the future terrorist groups may focus upon the use of "computer viruses" and falsification of bank records to essentially immobilize many industries in the developed countries. Media coverage of politically determined events often plays into the hands of terrorists. Although terrorist acts are generally viewed pejoratively today, past history is not consonant with this perception. From one perspective, it may be said that the perception of violence frequently lies in the eye of the beholder. Perception is functionally selective; motives differ. One person's terrorist is another person's hero, or, as it is often stated, "one man's terrorist is another man's freedom fighter."

Similar to the term *guerrilla*, from the French word *guerre* (war), terrorism has both positive and negative connotations. Violent incidents against person or property vary with religion, geography, political state, and the personal and psychological needs of the perpetrators. Throughout history numerous lives have been taken *en masse* in the name of some putative worthy cause or altruistic belief. In the time of Robespierre during the "reign of terror" in France in 1793–1794 the Jacobins characterized their activities as being entirely positive. Various other activist groups, principally the Girondins, became involved in widespread massacres.

Despite the fact that this period in history covered a relatively short span of a few months, several thousand persons were executed as a result of rebellious acts. Motivation rooted in such zealotry is more likely to be carried out by groups than on an individual basis.

Although the political aftermath of such events has been addressed at length by historians and political scientists, their psychological and physiological implications have received little or no systematic study. The term "terror" has both Greek and Latin roots, deriving from mythology. The two horses attached to the chariot of Aries or Mars, the Greek God of War, were named *Phobos* (terror or phobia) and *Deimos* (dread). The Latin root comes from the word *terrere* (to terrorize or frighten). Evil and danger are implied in any case.

Defining terrorism is not a simple matter because it is open to a variety of views. Arbitrarily, however, it may be defined by its political, psychological, and legal dimensions. A Vice Presidential Task Force defined terrorism as follows:

> [Terrorism is] the unlawful use or threat of violence against persons or property to further political or social objectives. It is generally intended to intimidate or coerce a government, individuals or groups to modify their behavior or policies. The terrorist's methods may include hostage-taking, aircraft piracy or sabotage, assassination, threats, hoaxes, indiscriminate bombings or shootings. (Vice President's Task Force on Terrorism, 1986)

Terrorism may be carried out as a government-sponsored undertaking or by private individuals and groups. Individual terrorism is often impulsive and disorganized, whereas group acts, even in non-state-sponsored terrorism, are often surprisingly well arranged and have motives similar to those which are underwritten by a government.

An important dichotomy exists with respect to individual versus group terrorism. Participants in group terrorism are calculating, thoughtful, and less likely to suffer from a definable emotional or mental disturbance; on the other hand, violent acts by a single perpetrator often lack real forethought and planning.

It is naive and unwise to regard most group terrorist as mentally ill. Moreover, this perception does a marked disservice to the victims. It can be a tragic mistake to devalue the terrorist and underestimate their emotional and mental capabilities. In the author's experience, terrorists are often highly intelligent and quite capable of "passing" a mental status examination with flying colors.

When emotions and feelings are involved, both physiological and psychological factors must be addressed in diagnosis and treatment. Fear is a primitive physiological response mediated by the sympathetic or thoracico-lumbar section of the autonomic nervous system via adrenergic impulses to the vital organs. It is a powerful motivator that is effectively played upon by knowledgeable perpetrators.

Since many young terrorists have led rather pathetic lives they become vulnerable, ready targets for recruitment into terrorist activities by avaricious leaders. Abu Nidal, for instance, considered by many as the arch-terrorist of recent times, has no difficulty whatever in recruiting young men willing to sacrifice themselves to his cause. This provides them with an identity and a vicarious feeling of personal power they never had themselves. It inculcates a misguided sense of importance and self-worth.

Terrorism, violence, and torture are often intertwined. *Violence* is defined as "the interhuman infliction of significant and avoidable pain and suffering" (Van Geuns, 1983, p. 11). In an effort to be succinct in the conference proceedings Vans Geuns did not elaborate upon intent by the use of such terms as "deliberate," "without consent," and "unacceptable to the victim." However, these terms are stated as implicit elsewhere in the proceedings. *Torture* has been defined as "the deliberate infliction of pain by one person upon another in an attempt to break down the will of the victim" (Stover & Nightingale, 1985, p. 4). In truncated form, this definition captures the essence of a statement on torture by the United Nations.

Participation in acts of torture by physicians and other health personnel is addressed by Stover & Nightingale (1985), who note that recorded instances of medical complicity in torture date back to 1532. Many anecdotal accounts were difficult to document prior to World War II, when German and Japanese physicians performed heinous atrocities under the guise of medical research. For example, Japanese physicians injected prisoners with bubonic plague, syphilis, cholera, and other deadly disease germs to ascertain the resistance of various nationalities and races to disease.

Stover and Nightingale (1985) refer to Amnesty International reports of medical personnel who tortured persons sentenced to prison for so-called political and criminal offenses. In 1980, the hands of four men were amputated by physicians or their assistants without anesthetic in Mauritania, despite protests from the local medical association. Reports were taken of Iranian medical personnel who drained the blood from their prisoners prior to execution for use with their own fighting forces in the Iran-Iraq war.

In the author's personal experience in treating former U.S. prisoners of war (POWs) from World War II, it is unmistakable that surgical procedures were carried out upon wounded prisoners without anesthetic. Although POWs were slapped and maltreated during surgery—an action explained by the Germans as necessary due to shortages of medical supplies. The Japanese employed various forms of torture and maltreatment with POW patients of mine from the Pacific theatre, torture including excising thumbnails with pliers, burning the back of the neck with cigarettes, placing a pole behind the knees and forcing knee bends until the knee joints were broken, throwing chunks of coal at the testicles of POWs working in coal mines, beatings with sticks, fists, and rifle butts, and confining selected victims to a box in the sun with little or no food and water until death ensued from extreme heat and dehydration. Such measures were designed to bring about conformity to rules and respect for existing authority.

Numerous accounts of brutality and torture were brought to my attention during my sojourns to Israel and the Middle East. An Israeli military physician told me that Israeli soldiers were especially fearful of being captured by the Syrians because of their brutality and torture. He stated that some Israeli soldiers carried lethal medication with them which they could ingest quickly rather than risk being captured by dreaded Syrian contingents. He spoke of an incident with which he was familiar concerning a young Syrian male who was publicly brutalized, tortured, and executed. The young man was discovered with a pair of sneakers which bore a mark indicating that they had been made in Israel. He was subsequently drawn and quartered in a public square for all to witness. Both arms and legs were attached to each of four separate vehicles which then dismembered his body by simultaneously pulling the limbs apart. This anecdote illustrated the heartless, barbarous measures which the Syrians could take against anyone, including their own citizens, for acts that were deemed to be patently incongruent with their own beliefs.

I was once asked to examine an American who had suffered brutal treatment and was discharged by his employer in an Arabic country. He had purchased a small prayer rug while on holiday in a nearby country. Upon his return he was asked to give the customs officer many dollars worth of *bahksheesh*, or Arabic money, in order to be allowed to keep the rug. He refused and stated that he would mail the rug back to the United States rather than pay an exorbitant amount to keep it in his possession.

One of the customs officers then falsely accused him of attempting to bring hashish back into this Arabic country where he worked. He was then taken to a separate room, interrogated, and maltreated in order to force a confession with respect to the hashish. He became fearful that he would be raped, since he had witnessed the guards assaulting other prisoners. When he could no longer stand up after his knee joints were broken, a pole was placed between his legs with a guard on each end and lifted upward mashing his testicles. Months of brutality followed in a prison cell where he slept on the floor with no toilet facilities, able to wipe himself only with his hands. The putrefaction of his own decaying feces and that of other prisoners was overwhelming.

Allodi and Cowgill, (1982) detail specific aspects of torture in South America. Methods of torture included such techniques as beatings, electricity applied to the genitals and other parts of the body, stretching, submersion of a victim's head in mixtures of vomit, blood, feces, and urine, burns, suspension, rape and other sexual torture, boxing the ears, and being forced to stand with outstretched arms holding weights for hours and days. Numerous ongoing physical and psychological sequelae frequently follow these tortures, particularly disorders of the skin and joints, dysfunction of various body organs, anxiety, phobias, and depression.

## GEOGRAPHIC PHENOMENA

Despite the publicity surrounding terrorist acts, the United States has been subjected to very little international terrorism. Most terrorist acts in the late 1970s and early 1980s occurred in Western Europe, with a large number also taking place in Latin America. Western Europe was a primary target for such activity, even though it originated in the Middle East. As the reader may see from Table 7.1, 57% of the terrorist activity in 1977 occurred in Western Europe, fostering greater psychological impact and extensive media coverage when such activity occurs in modern developed countries. A decade later a marked reversal developed in favor of the Middle East, which accounts for nearly half of these terrorist incidents.

Terrorist acts of Middle East origin increased 178% in the decade from 1978 and 1987. One of every four terrorist acts in Western Europe during 1985–86 originated in the Middle East. The types of attacks are worthy of note. Much press and media coverage focuses upon terrorist acts against Americans, in point of fact, during 1987 only 18% of terrorist incidents involved American citizens. Israel has endured more casualties

**TABLE 7.1  Percentage of International Terrorist Incidents by World Regions, 1977 and 1987***

|  | 1977 | 1987 |
|---|---|---|
| Africa | 6.0 | 3.0 |
| Asia | 3.0 | 20.09 |
| Eastern Europe | 1.0 | .01 |
| Latin America | 15.0 | 13.0 |
| Middle East | 11.0 | 45.0 |
| North America | 7.0 | -0- |
| Western Europe | 57.0 | 18.0 |
|  | 100.0 | 100.00 |

*Percentages computed by the author from data provided by the Office of the Ambassador at Large for Counterterrorism, U.S. Department of State, 1989.

than the United States, which is significant in view of the vast population differences between the two countries. Since 1983, when 41% of these incidents involved U.S. citizens, the number has declined sharply. In general, Western Europe has suffered the greatest number of incidents. Bombings account for more than half of all terrorist actions. This figure exceeds armed attacks, the second leading method used by terrorists, by more than two and a half times. This frequency is nearly four times that of the third leading cause; namely, arson. Table 7.2 shows that bombings occur more often than all other methods combined.

This is partially attributable to the fact that bombings exert a telling effect and can be carried out in a "hit-and-run" manner. Persons engaged in bombings are less likely to be apprehended and do not have to devote

**TABLE 7.2  International Terrorist Incidents, 1978–1987***

|  | N | Percentage |
|---|---|---|
| Armed Attacks | 1,214 | 20.0 |
| Arson | 831 | 14.0 |
| Barricade, Hostages | 90 | 2.0 |
| Barricade, No Hostages | 84 | 1.0 |
| Bombings | 3,191 | 54.0 |
| Skyjackings | 64 | 1.0 |
| Kidnappings | 426 | 7.0 |
| Sabotage/Vandalism | 68 | 1.0 |
|  | 5,968 | 100.0 |

*Percentages rounded and computed by the author from data provided by the Office of the Ambassador at Large for Counterterrorism, U.S. Department of State, 1989.

**TABLE 7.3  Casualties from International Terrorism, Decade 1978–1987\***

| International | N | Percent |
|---|---|---|
| Dead | 4,925 | 30.0 |
| Wounded | 11,253 | 70.0 |
| Total Casualties | 16,178 | 100.0 |

| United States | N | Percent |
|---|---|---|
| Dead | 387 | 41.0 |
| Wounded | 560 | 59.0 |
| Total Casualties | 947 | 100.0 |

\*Percentages computed by the author from data provided by the Office of the Ambassador at Large for Counterterrorism, U.S. Department of State, 1989.

time to guarding their victims. The experience of Pan American Flight 103 on December 21, 1988, is a cardinal example of the effects of bombing. Terrorists kidnapped and held persons hostage in sufficient numbers to heighten psychological warfare and media coverage while still remaining sufficiently unencumbered to be able to promote other terrorist activities as well. Moreover, when a group has a wish to emphasize or punctuate a particular message, a kidnapping or hostage-taking incursion provides a dramatic means for doing so. The fact that the U.S. has suffered fewer casualties than most countries does not lessen its impact, especially upon surviving victims. The high value placed upon human life by the Western World reinforces the usefulness of hostage-taking to the terrorists. The psychic pain and suffering endured by friends and family members nurtures the perpetrator's psychological warfare tactics. Although U.S. casualties during the decade from 1978–1987 numbered slightly less than 6% of the total, the psychic trauma of those involved was often severe and lasting. Moreover, as shown in Table 7.3, the percentage of persons dead among incidents involving U.S. citizens exceeds international figures substantially, 41% to 30%. Table 7.4 shows the preponderance of hostage victims from business and diplomatic circles.

## Precipitating Stress Factors and Related Protective Factors

As the author has noted elsewhere (Frederick, 1987), stress and coping issues have generated a number of theories, especially during the past two

**TABLE 7.4  International Terrorist Incidents By Victim Type and Facility 1978–1987\***

| International Victim/Facility | N | Percent |
| --- | --- | --- |
| Business | 1433 | 35 |
| Diplomat | 1465 | 36 |
| Government | 599 | 15 |
| Military | 582 | 14 |
| | 4079 | 100 |

| Against U.S. Victim/Facility | N | Percent |
| --- | --- | --- |
| Business | 565 | 42 |
| Diplomat | 302 | 22 |
| Government | 184 | 14 |
| Military | 304 | 22 |
| | 1355 | 100 |

\*Figures computed by the author from data provided by the Office of the Ambassador at Large for Counterterrorism, U.S. Department of State, 1989.

decades. The literature is quite varied due to the approaches taken by investigators from different disciplines. Early authors addressed the topic of stress from three perspectives; anthropological (Cannon, 1932), biological (Selye, 1952), and psychological (Janis, 1971). Moreover, the influence of biochemical, genetic, environmental, and interpersonal stress variables has been shown to contribute to violent behavior (Asterita, 1985; Burrowes, Hales, & Arrington, 1988; Hogben & Cornfield, 1961; Modlin, 1986; Sonnenberg, 1988). Coping with stress may be enhanced or lessened through biochemical routes. The differences between victims who develop post-traumatic stress and those who do not are elusive, and those victims who do not continue to require further study. Nevertheless, we do know that coping styles differ with personality structure, type of stress, and supportive resources. Fields (1976) has shown that entire societies can become trauma victims.

Leopold and Dillon (1963) indicate that intense stress, even for a relatively short period of time, can evoke deleterious physiological and psychological sequelae. Over a prolonged period it can evoke hypertension and adrenal failure and wreak havoc with the autonomic nervous system. The heart, brain, kidneys, and eyes become vital target organs. Impairment of these organs produces further stress and psychic trauma, resulting in a vicious cycle.

Phobic symptoms following severe trauma may cause individuals to believe that they are going to die; these symptoms can become disabling to the point of virtual emotional paralysis. Autonomic nervous system responses, such as startle reactions and tachycardia, are cardinal components of post-traumatic stress disorder. Poor judgment, loss of concentration, loss of libido, social withdrawal, self-destructive behavior, memory disturbances, and confusion may obtain in varying degrees.

The coping mechanism is an integral part of past experience. The ordeal of captivity "does not always end with freedom," as former hostage David Jacobsen notes in his book *Hostages: My Nightmare in Beirut* (1991). Father Lawrence Martin Jenco, one of a number of former hostages, with whom the author has interacted or worked, has shared the feeling that complete freedom can only come when all other hostages are free and a resolution is reached within the self with respect to emotional conflicts. Some persons are strong-willed and assertive, others are more introversive and less overtly assertive. Any coping style must be respected, since each person has the right to cope in a fashion most suited for themselves. For example, Father Jenco relied upon his deep religious beliefs, while David Jacobsen and others placed greater emphasis upon exercise and physical conditioning.

The author has found salient stress factors and related protective factors to include: 1) severity of stressor; 2) restriction of movement; 3) being alone during confinement; 4) age; 5) support systems during and following captivity; 6) duration of stress; 7) physical environment; and 8) premorbid vulnerability. By and large, strong positive correlations result in more severe stress reactions with the first four conditions noted, except for age; moderate positive correlations occur in the presence of the latter four factors. An exception is the age factor. Persons over 40 years old generally fare better and develop fewer psychological problems than those under 40. Life experience seems to exert a salutary protective effect in diminishing disabling fears.

The author's research reveals further that the following coping factors consistently provide protection against stress among persons who have experienced being held hostage: 1) belief in the inner strength of the self; 2) reflective thoughts of loved ones; 3) faith in some superordinate power; 4) continuing hope that captivity will end favorably; 5) use of one's powers of calculation to interact and plan for escape or release; 6) physical and mental exercise; 7) appropriate expression of anger; and 8) ability to focus attention and become task-oriented.

Stress cannot be measured or defined without considering both stressor and "stressee." Stress cannot exist without a host upon which to act. Coping can appear as a passive or indifferent response. Furthermore, stress must be per-

| Independent Variable | Intervening Variable | Dependent Variable |
|---|---|---|
| Psychological Stressors | Person/Host | Condition |
| Trauma/ Stressor | No PF/Stress ---▶Viable stresses -----▶ PTSD | |
| | PF/No stress --▶No viable stresses-▶No PTSD | |
| Public Health Stressors | | |
| Pneumocystis carinii/ Stressor | No PF T4 cells ---▶ Viable Host -----▶Disease | |
| | PF T4 cells -----▶No viable Host--▶No Disease | |

PF= Protective Factors

**FIGURE 7.1** Protective Factors Trauma/Stress Model For Psychological and Public Health Stressors.

sonal. The energy that goes into managing or controlling it is an implicit part of stress itself. Stress is analogous to bacteria in the field of public health: a stressor, like a bacteria pest, virus, must find an acceptable host for disease (stress) to take hold. If one resists or becomes immune to the pest (stressor) then neither stress nor a viable host (stressee) will be present. A condition of immunity produces a negative host. Thus, both prevention and treatment must be targeted toward the heart of the issue (Frederick, 1989).

Psychological immunization, similarly termed "psychological inoculation" (Cameron & Meichenbaum, 1982; Meichenbaum, 1977) and "incident-specific" treatment (Frederick, 1986) are both directed toward amelioration of stress problems in a vulnerable host. The latter approach, in particular, underscores the value of healthy ego strength and deemphasizes the sick role.

## DIAGNOSTIC AND TREATMENT CONSIDERATIONS

### Diagnosis

A number of stressors are likely to evoke some form of psychic trauma. While similarities in symptom formation occur, there are appreciable differences as well. There appears to be a current tendency, at least in the

United States, to label virtually every psychological reaction to a severe stressor as a post-traumatic stress disorder (PTSD). The proliferation of compensation claims by Vietnam War veterans has added impetus to this phenomenon. Curiously, this diagnostic classification is both overused and underused. Such misuse results in cases being missed where PTSD exists, while in other instances the term is employed where it does not belong. A multitude of inappropriate symptoms are perpetuated in the name of PTSD; it is the diagnosis of the decade. In large measure, this is due to the fact that a litany of symptoms found in other disorders overlap or resemble those seen in PTSD (American Psychiatric Association, 1987).

Psychic trauma does not invariably elicit post-traumatic stress disorder. Among the common diagnostic entities with which PTSD is confused are phobic disorder, depressive reactions, generalized anxiety disorder, borderline disorder, and dissociative reaction (psychogenic amnesia).

Elements of each of these disorders may manifest themselves in PTSD, which only emphasizes the necessity for astute clinical acumen in this highly specialized area. Every clinician who diagnoses and treats patients needs explicit training and experience with such cases. Moreover, research experience with trauma subjects can prove to be of great value. As in depression, for example, sleep disorders, eating disturbances, marked diminished interest in activities, fatigue, difficulty in concentration, inappropriate guilt, and loss of libido also often occur in PTSD. Likewise, PTSD resembles simple phobia; symptoms of distress from a specific stimulus, interference with work ability, and recognition that the fear is unreasonable occur in both disorders. However, in phobia, as opposed to PTSD, the phobic stimulus is unrelated to trauma content. The motor tension, autonomic nervous system hyperactivity, excessive vigilance, and scanning which are present in generalized anxiety disorder are also frequently seen in PTSD. Since PTSD patients can be irritable and appear irrational, they may be confused with a borderline diagnosis. While dissociative-like behavior may appear in PTSD, it is by no means universal, but the presence of anxiety is unmistakable. Eidetic dreams occur with PTSD while oneiric dreams occur in other disorders. In addition, Axis II diagnoses, such as substance abuse, are increasingly present in PTSD subjects, which contribute to an already caliginous picture.

Care must be taken to examine the patient fully while obtaining a medical, social, and family history. In the author's view, it is impossible to diagnose an individual accurately who has experienced psychic trauma without taking physiological measures such as pulse rate and blood pressure readings, along with an appropriate battery of psychological tests. As noted by Dalton, Garter,

**TABLE 7.5  Reaction Index Severity Levels for Subjects Experiencing Different Stressors**

| Groups | N | Doubtful | Mild | Moderate | Severe | Very Severe |
|---|---|---|---|---|---|---|
| POWs | 50 | 4 | 7 | 14 | 17 | 8 |
| Physical Assault Victims | 58 | 5 | 9 | 18 | 14 | 4 |
| Disaster Victims | 100 | 11 | 19 | 42 | 21 | 7 |
| Hostages | 50 | 2 | 5 | 10 | 19 | 14 |
| Rape Victims | 50 | 3 | 6 | 12 | 16 | 11 |

Pearson Chi Square = 28.97; $df$ = 16; $p$ = .02

After Frederick, C. J. (1987). Psychic trauma in victims or crime and terrorism. In G. R. VandenBos & B. K. Bryant (Eds.), *Cataclysms, crises, and catastrophes* (p. 74). Washington, DC: American Psychological Association.

Lips, & Ryan (1986) and Frederick (1987) the following comprise an appropriate psychological test battery: personality test, mood disorder scale, assessment of intellectual functioning, neuropsychologicals, and measure of psychic trauma and anxiety. While other tests may suffice, those recommended here represent a distillation of the experiences of a number of clinicians who have worked extensively with PTSD populations.

The validation of unsettling thoughts and experiences via cardiovascular measures is essential. Trouble spots can be located and highlighted for purposes of both diagnosis and treatment. In some instances, areas of psychic disturbance occur through symbolic association, which are not consciously recognized by the victim. Such problems are not palpable through standard clinical interviews. Sampling areas of genuine psychic trauma will often elicit increased readings in pulse rate and blood pressure of 20 points or more. The possibility of separating out a factitious disorder or malingering is increased immeasurably, no matter how skilled the examiner, through the use of physiological measures to complement the interviews and psychological tests employed. Since these procedures are noninvasive, when appropriately used, they can enhance the patient's confidence in the examiner. In addition, responses to severe trauma correlate significantly with Reaction Index scores (Frederick, 1987).

## Treatment

Traditional methods are unsatisfactory in alleviating the symptoms of severe psychic trauma. Customary treatment procedures seldom suffice, including the usual crisis intervention support practices. In cases where severe psychic trauma has occurred, e.g., hostage-taking, rape, physical assault, airplane crashes, child abuse, and many catastrophic disasters, specific treatment must be skillfully employed or the victim may never resolve the trauma or function with appropriate emotional and mental efficiency.

I am convinced that treatment should consist of the following components (Frederick, 1990a, 1990b):

1) *Initial supportive psychotherapy*. Therapy supplies reassurance and reestablishes lost trust.

2) *Relaxation instruction*. This provides needed tension reduction and prepares the individual for other procedures that follow.

3) *Recounting of specific incidents*. Reviewing unsettling scenes during a state of relaxation assists in tolerating provocative stimuli.

4) *Slow motion focusing*. Elements of distress are reworked and reduced in strength.

5) *Correlating*. Anxiety-provoking stimuli are related to other significant facets of the patient's life.

6) *Deconditioning*. Troublesome autonomic nervous system arousal responses are reduced via biofeedback-like techniques.

7) *In vitro and in vivo techniques*. Traumatic events are treated first in the laboratory/office and then in life or simulated in-life scenes.

8) *Psychological reaction indices*. Reaction Index tests during and after treatment objectively measure initial and residual PTSD.

In this author's experience, most persons subjected to major traumatic events find it difficult to maintain mental and emotional equilibrium in executing their daily activities in the absence of treatment. Moreover, it is of utmost importance for clinicians to receive direct experience and training with victims. Most responses by victims should be viewed as normal reactions experienced by normal people. Thus, such a specialized area of mental health practice requires sensitivity and flexibility to avoid disconsonance with those who have experienced dehumanizing ordeals. Former hostages may appear to be very touchy and feel exploited, especially by health professionals and the media. Re-establishing personal confidence is of paramount importance.

Apart from the works of a few investigators, such as those reported by the author (Frederick, 1983, 1987, 1990b), the bulk of the subjects studied in terms of both diagnosis and treatment of post-traumatic stress disorder (PTSD) have been Vietnam combat veterans. Variations of behavior therapy, principally desensitization, combined with some form of individual or group therapy have constituted the majority of treatment modalities. The author (Frederick, 1987), however, has emphasized the importance of physiological measures and incident-specific treatment as a *sine qua non* for trauma mastery.

Among the newer therapeutic procedures presumed to be of immediate benefit to persons suffering from PTSD is so-called eye movement desensitization (EMD) therapy (Puk, 1991; Shapiro, 1989a, 1989b, 1991; Wolpe & Abrams, 1991). This procedure consists of a series of saccadic eye movements while the patient holds the head steady and maintains a mentally distressing image of the unsettling traumatic event. These eye movements are induced by following the therapist's finger or other object laterally with the eyes back and forth at the rate of one per second in sets of 20 to 30 with further repetitions as needed. Distressing images and attending symptoms such as nightmares are said to have been rapidly defused or eliminated in selected cases.

The long-term efficacy and applicability of EMD treatment to a broad range of trauma stressors remains to be shown. The investigations by Shapiro (1989, 1991a, 1991b), Puk (1991), Wolpe and Abrams (1991), already noted, have focused upon subjects who reported experiencing sexual abuse or Vietnam combat.

Although dramatically appealing, physiological and psychological measures of positive change and reduction of emotional response to traumatic events as a result of EMD therapy have not been demonstrated. Furthermore, no substantial explanation of the physiology of EMD has been forthcoming to date. The subject's memory of the event seems to have been changed, which alters the perception of it. EMD may serve as a distraction device or effect a temporary diminution of the retention of symptoms in selected cases. However, if the many positive anecdotal experiences reported prove worthwhile after careful scrutiny, a major contribution to treatment will have been made.

In a related vein, there is a plethora of cases in which childhood sexual abuse is presumed to have been present when none existed. Some improvident therapists become imbued with the notion that if a given form of anxiety or dissociative reaction is present, childhood sexual abuse must have occurred. The therapist then goes about convincing the subject that he/she must be repressing such an event which, in turn, stimulates dreams and fantasies of a similar kind. Following termination of treatment, it may take the "victim" years to unravel these associations and recognize that the event in question either did not occur at all or did not occur in the traumatic form elicited by the therapist's comments. Shapiro

(1991) admits that in unskilled and untrained hands, under EMD therapy, patients are placed at risk of inducing "ocular problems, re-traumatization, suicidal reactions, etc." (p. 136). Indeed, all therapists would do well to remember the physician's code to *do no harm*. In order for its efficacy to be more real than apparent, EMD treatment of psychic trauma will require much further study and documentation. As with all procedures, it must meet necessary and sufficient conditions for careful controls of subjects, methods of presentation, and various kinds of stressors over an appreciable period of time.

It is quite threatening to hostages and torture victims to feel that they need psychological help. It adds to their self-doubt and poor self-esteem. They may be reluctant to talk much about their ordeal. Since they have a great need to convince themselves that they are intact emotionally and mentally, a damaged self-concept may be inadvertently reinforced by insensitive mental health treatment. Once hostages are released from captivity, unrealistic expectations often develop. Unrealistically, victims may expect benevolence from others and joy within themselves, the bulk of the time. The author has seen numerous instances where inappropriate treatment for psychic trauma has brought deleterious results. Unfortunately, many naive but well-intentioned therapists are untrained and inexperienced in treating serious psychic trauma cases. In view of these shortcomings, they may actually be harmful to the patient and turn him or her away from treatment and materially delay recovery. It is imperative to create a therapeutic climate wherein victims are allowed to experience any feeling, doubt, or criticism they may have of their environment as they perceive it. Anger is difficult to tolerate for the victim and covictim family members but its expression is frequently critical to trauma mastery. Whatever strengthens the damaged ego and self-concept serves as a benchmark for psychic reconstruction. Ego reinforcement is central to recovery. The incident-specific components of treatment protocol are a *sine qua non* for trauma mastery.

## Children and Family as Covictims

Involving family members in treatment, both individually and together, can be of inestimable value. However, this process must be handled with special sensitivity to avoid heightening defensiveness and feelings of denigration while enhancing cooperation and self-worth.

In principle, the same techniques and caveats applicable to adults apply to the children and family members of victims as well. Eth and Pynoos

(1985) and Pynoos et al., (1987) studied children subjected to traumatic situations, including an assassination. The degree of direct exposure to the stimulus and support networks were important factors relating to trauma severity and recovery rate over time. Milgram (1982) has reported impressive work with Israeli children and youth subjected to war-related stress.

## Principles of Intervention

Early intervention with traumatic victims offers an important opportunity to mitigate some of the deleterious effects. The wording and demeanor of the clinician must be adjusted to the person and circumstances. In essence, the following comments should be made to victims at the outset:

1) I am sorry this happened;
2) I am glad you are allright (or ''I am glad you are going to be allright);
3) It was not your fault;
4) I am going to be here for you (or ''someone will be here for you'').

These comments have been adapted in the work from those noted by Symonds (1980). This approach can be of inestimable value in precluding any ''second injury'' or gratuitous trauma imposed by insensitive authority figures or other persons in the victim's immediate life space.

Various tension reduction procedures have been employed effectively by some victims, on occasion, without their having being taught. There is little doubt that prior knowledge of such techniques can be most useful during periods of prolonged stress. William F. Niehous, an American business executive who was held hostage in South America, offers these suggestions for potential victims: engage in active forms of communication with captors on nonthreatening topics; attempt to convince captors to recognize the victim as a human being rather than an object; set personal goals for oneself; attend to personal health—eat and exercise; and maintain faith in something outside oneself (Niehous, 1985).

Weisaeth (1989) reported that of 13 Norwegian sailors who were tortured after being taken hostage near the coast of Libya in 1984 ''not a single seaman gave in to the torture'' (p. 63). However, 7 of the 13 developed PTSD, whereas 6 did not. Although not marked enough to warrant a diagnosis, some psychological symptoms appeared in virtually all subjects. Differences between subjects with clear psychological distress versus those without such symptoms appeared to be determined by 1) premorbid vulnerability; 2) absence of productive routine work during captivity; and 3) severity of the experience.

## Faith

Faith in some superordinate power beyond the self has been reported as a protective factor in varying degrees by virtually all of the numerous hostages with whom the author has interacted. This may or may not take the form of classical religion, although some organizational structure often manifests itself. This phenomenon is found in both the primary hostage victim and family member covictims alike. Inasmuch as the core of victimization is the loss of personal power over oneself with no viable options apparent, it is quite logical that the victim turns to something superordinate as a self-protective, tension-reducing measure. Lack of appreciation of the victim's need at such a time may constitute a contretemps which can come back to haunt the insensitive intervenor. The thought that the situation is out of one's own control results in helplessness followed by hopelessness. At that point, one may become suicidal or engage in a belief beyond the existing circumstances in order to extricate oneself from a seemingly insoluble dilemma. With most persons who are essentially healthy emotionally and physically, faith can become a valuable adjunct to the ego defense structure. Psychologically, a basic function of faith and religious beliefs is to reduce anxiety. However, such a process may be partially dependent upon premorbid vulnerability. One Roman Catholic chaplain told me that several chaplains from various denominations left the clergy after their stressful and heart-rending experiences in Vietnam.

Curiously, my colleagues in the Middle East have emphasized that faith comprises the nucleus of effective mental health treatment. *In Challah Bukrah, Malesh* is a phrase used in the Middle East; broadly translated, this phrase means that worry is for naught because Allah must take care of matters. Faith offers a useful buffer against tragedy and the inevitability of death.

None of the emotional reactions to trauma is abnormal, per se; it is only when the person feels dysfunctional or becomes ineffective in work or social relations that ordinary prudence perforce descries the need for intervention. Needless worry is often precipitated by instant experts and overly eager therapists. Although it is wise to recognize that it is healthy and commendable to address a problem before it worsens and becomes chronic, it is not always easy to do this after suffering severe trauma. Individual feelings should always be respected, and the decision to engage in treatment must be left to the victim. In such cases it is usually prudent to be wary of overusage of psychoactive drugs. Some studies have suggested that severely distressed persons may profit from medication, while mildly distressed individuals frequently do not (Modlin, 1986).

In summary, psychophysiological measures, such as pulse rate and blood pressure, coupled with incident-specific therapy have been most fruitful. The author has found that focusing upon disturbing stimuli in slow motion while in a relaxed state has been enormously successful in both diagnosis and treatment of severe cases of psychic trauma. This process is accompanied by psychotherapy in order to unravel and resolve past associative experiences and their negative residuals which may be related to the present distress. It must be remembered that the body and mind possess a natural urge for healing themselves. This process must always be enhanced and never compromised. All of our noteworthy advances in science and medicine must be cast against the backdrop of understanding the human condition. This may well constitute the most important aspect of professional endeavor. Faith in the strength and resiliency of the human spirit should never be forgotten or underestimated. The sustaining power of understanding must accompany wisdom. Irrespective of one's religious beliefs, the book of Proverbs provides rich food for thought:

> *For the Lord by his wisdom hath created the earth but by understanding hath he established the heavens.* (Proverbs, 3:19)

# REFERENCES

Allodi, F., & Cogwill, G. (1981). "Ethical and psychiatric aspects of torture: A Canadian Study." *Canadian Journal of Psychiatry, 27*, 98–102.

American Psychiatric Association. (1987). *Diagnostic and statistical manual of mental disorders*. (3rd ed.). Washington, DC: Author.

Arnold, T. E., & Kennedy, M. (1988). Think about terrorism: The new warfare. New York: Walker and Company.

Asterita, M. E. (1985). *The physiology of stress*. New York: Human Sciences Press.

Burrowes, K. L., Hales, R. E., & Arrington, E. (1988). Research on the biologic aspects of violence. *The psychiatric clinics of North America* (581–589).

Cameron, R., & Meichenbaum, D. (1982). The nature of effective coping and the treatment of stress related problems: A cognitive-behavioral perspective. In L. Goldberg & S. Breznitz (Eds.), *Handbook of stress* (pp. 695–71). New York: The Free Press.

Cannon, W. B. (1942). Voodoo death. *American Anthropologist, 44*, 169–181.

Dalton, J. E., Garter, S. H., Lips, O. J., & Ryan, J. J. (1986). Psychological assessment instrument in PTSD treatment problems. *VA Practitioner 8*, 41–51.

Eth, S., & Pynoos, R. S. (1985). Post-traumatic stress disorder in children. Washington, DC: American Psychiatric Press, Inc.

Fields, R. M. (1976). *Society under siege*. Philadelphia: Temple University Press.

Frederick, C. J. (1983). Violence and disasters: Immediate and long-term consequences. In H. A. Van Geuns (Ed.), *Helping victims of violence* (pp. 32–46). The Hague, Netherlands: Ministry of Welfare, Health, and Cultural Affairs.

Frederick, C. J. (1985). Children traumatized by catastrophic situations. In S. Eth & R. S. Pynoos (Eds.), *Post-traumatic stress disorder in children* (pp. 73–99). Washington, DC. American Psychiatric Press.

Frederick, C. J. (1986). Treatment for post-traumatic stress disorder: An incident-specific approach. In M. J. Goldstein, B. Baker, & K. R. Jamison (Eds.), *Abnormal psychology* (pp. 465–468). Boston: Little, Brown.

Frederick, C. J. (1987). Psychic trauma in victims of crime and terrorism. In G. R. Vandenbos & B. K. Bryant (Eds.), *Cataclysms, crises and catastrophes: Psychology in action* (pp. 55–108). Washington, DC: American Psychological Association.

Frederick, C. J. (1990a). Resourcefulness in coping with severe trauma: The case of the hostages. In M. Rosenbaum (Ed.), *Learned resourcefulness: On coping skills, self control and adaptive behavior* (pp. 218–228). New York: Springer Publishing Co.

Frederick, C. J. (1990b). Diagnosis and treatment of post traumatic stress disorder. In A. D. Manglesdorf. *Proceedings Seventh Users Workshop: Training for psychic trauma*, Report #91–001 (pp. 35–39). San Antonio, U.S. Army Health Services Command.

Hogben, G. I., & Cornfield, R. B. (1961). Treatment of traumatic war neuroses with phenelzine. *Archives of general psychiatry, 38*, 440–445.

Jacobsen, D. (1991). *Hostage. My nightmare in Beirut*. New York: Donald Fine.

Janis, I. L. (1971). *Stress and frustration*. New York: Harcourt.

Leopold, R. L., & Dillon, H., (1963). Psycho-anatomy of disaster. *American Journal of Psychiatry, 119*, 913–921.

Meichenbaum, D. (1977). *Cognitive-behavior modification: An integrative approach*. New York: Plenum.

Milgram, N. A. (1982). War related stress in Israeli children and youth. In L. Goldberger & S. Breznitz (Eds.), *Handbook of stress: Theoretical and clinical aspects* (pp. 656–676). New York: The Free Press.

Modlin, H. C. (1986). Post traumatic stress disorder: No longer just for war veterans. *Post Graduate Medicine, 70*, 26–44.

Niehous, W. F. (1985). Surviving captivity: II. The hostage's point of view. In B. M. Jenkins (Ed.), *Terrorism and personal protection* (pp. 423–433). Stoneham, MA: Butterworth Publishers.

Puk, G. (1991). Treating traumatic memories: A case report on the eye movement desensitization procedure. *Journal of Behavioral Therapy and Experimental Psychiatry, 22*, 149–151.

Pynoos, R. S., Frederick, C. J., Nader, K., Arroyo, W., Steinberg, A., Eth, S., Nunez, F., & Fairbanks, L. (1987). Life threat and post traumatic stress in school age children. *Archives of General Psychiatry, 44*.

Selye, H. (1952). *The story of the Adaptation Syndrome* Montreal: Acta.

Shapiro, F. (1989a). Efficacy of the eye movement desensitization procedure in the treatment of traumatic memories. *Journal of Traumatic Stress, 2*, 199–223.

Shapiro, F. (1989b). Eye movement desensitization: A new treatment for post-traumatic stress disorder. *Journal of Behavior Therapy and Experimental Psychiatry, 20*, 211–217.

Shapiro, F. (1991). Eye movement desensitization & reprocessing procedure: From EMD to EMD/R—A new treatment model for anxiety and related trauma. *The Behavior Therapist, 14*, 133–136.

Stover, E., & Nightingale, E. (1985). *The breaking of bodies and minds* New York: W. H. Freeman.

Symonds, M. (1980). The "second injury" to victims. In L. Kivens (Ed.), *Evaluation and change: Services for survivors* (pp. 36–38). Minneapolis: Minneapolis Medical Research Foundation.

Van Geuns, H. A. (Ed.). (1983). Helping victims of violence. *Proceedings of a Working Group on the Psychosocial Consequences of Violence*, p. 11. The Hague Ministry of Welfare, The Hague, Netherlands: Health and Cultural Affairs.

Vice President's Task Force on Terrorism, Report. (1986).

Weisaeth, L. (1989). Torture of a Norwegian ship's crew: The torture, stress reactions and psychiatric after-effects. *Acta Psychiatrica Scandinavica, Supplementum 355*, 63–72.

Wolpe, J., & Abrams, J. (1991). Post-traumatic stress disorder overcome by eye movement desensitization: A case report. *Journal of Behavior Therapy and Experimental Psychiatry, 22*, 39–43.

# CHAPTER 8

# Stress and the Psychiatric Professional: Coping with the Practice of a Changing Profession and Strains from the Administrative Life

*Joel Yager and Milton Greenblatt*

## INTRODUCTION

STRESSORS affecting today's psychiatrists, stemming from forces both within and outside the profession in society at large, may be transforming psychiatry into a less desirable profession. The stressors acting on contemporary psychiatrist administrators may be even more pronounced than on other practitioners. As a complement to the "outer-directed" chapters in this volume, written by psychiatrists and psychologists dealing with their varied areas of stress-related clinical and research concerns, this chapter takes an inner-directed perspective. We address the stressors that the psychiatrist faces in two broad areas: first with respect to the changing profession as a whole, and then, as is appropriate in a volume honoring a great psychiatric administrator, Dr. Ransom Arthur, we will focus on the increasingly important role of the psychiatrist as administrator and leader. We will describe the sources of professional stressors currently impacting the profession; factors that contribute to the vulnerability of some psychiatrists to these stressors; suggestions regarding coping mechanisms and various "stress-protective factors" for general psychiatrists and psychiatrist administrators; and the counterbalancing rewards of professional lives in psychiatry and psychiatric administration. To amplify and illustrate how psychiatrists might adapt to a rapidly

Portions of this section were taken from Greenblatt, M. (1985). Administrative psychiatry. In H. I. Kaplan and B. Sadock (Eds.), *Comprehensive textbook of psychiatry: Vol. 4* (pp. 2007–2015). Baltimore, MD: Williams and Wilkins. See in particular "Reduction of administrative stress," p. 2014.

changing profession, we examine through a higher powered lens one illustrative type of psychiatric career—that of the psychiatric administrator. We use as examples the results of our research studies on the special case of those coping with a particularly demanding administrative role, that of State Commissioner of Mental Health. However, we suspect that the findings will evoke parallel experiences from Dr. Arthur's broad leadership experiences in Navy, Veterans Administration, and university organizations. Leadership roles in all these organizations deserve additional study in order to ascertain the extent to which our findings are generalizable.

## STRESSORS AFFECTING THE PSYCHIATRIC PROFESSION

### Stressors in General Psychiatry

The sense that careers in psychiatry may be the fact that perceived as increasingly stressful stems from several observations. First, the fact that the number of American medical students entering psychiatry has been falling sharply, off 18% in the past 4 years (Weissman, in press), has been taken to suggest an awareness of increasing stress in the profession. The reasons for the dropoff are undoubtedly complex and relate to issues of decreased work satisfaction, autonomy, and, for some, income.

Second, grumbling about career by psychiatric practitioners in professional and social settings is said to be increasing, with more pronounced expressions of dissatisfaction. Many remark that they would not recommend psychiatry as a profession for their children, because the profession is becoming too regulated, beset by too many hassles, and because psychiatry no longer seems to be what it used to be. An almost palpable, pervasive sense that the "good old days" have been lost forever appears increasingly to permeate the psychiatric zeitgeist.

Stressors challenging psychiatry include a variety of economic, social, interprofessional, and intraprofessional forces, as well as those imposed by mushrooming scientific advances. Psychiatrists who are most vulnerable to these changes include those whose professional niches and practice patterns afford greater direct exposure to the effects of the rapidly shifting economic, social, and scientific forces, and who lack sufficient personal flexibility to change their practices accordingly.

## 1. Pressures for medical cost containment

Pressures of industry and government have already resulted in dramatically shorter hospital stays with active utilization review, capitation programs in place of pass-through charges, increasing patient copayments to reduce utilization, gatekeeper programs that limit access to specialists, and other processes designed to cut costs, if not always ineffective or inefficient care.

The dramatically reduced lengths of stay have negatively affected what Rabkin (1982) has called the physician's SAG index (i.e., sense of anxiety vs. gratification). Now, with briefer and more complicated hospitalizations, psychiatrists feel more anxiety around their hospitalized patients, but no longer have as many days of professional gratification visiting patients as they recover in hospital. Furthermore, the reduced lengths of stay have also resulted in dropping psychiatric bed censuses in private for-profit and not-for-profit hospitals all around the nation, reducing the income of many psychiatrists for whom inpatient work constituted a significant part of practice.

Also, physicians' fees are among the costs to be contained. Resource-Based Relative Value Scales (RBRVS) for physician services (Shiao et al., 1988) are still being negotiated. Psychiatry will not gain much in contrast to primary care specialties, and in some respects may lose with this system. Indeed, Medicare payments for geriatric psychiatry have recently been cut back.

Furthermore, psychiatrists' anticipated incomes are already among the lowest in the medical profession, generally on a par with internal medicine and exceeding only those for family medicine and pediatrics. For heavily indebted students who are considering a career in psychiatry rather than one of the many more lucrative specialties, the cost-benefit ratio shifts in a negative direction.

## 2. Increasing indebtedness of medical students

The debts of $80,000 to $120,000 carried by many of today's housestaff are not inconsequential. Oryshkevich (1989) suggests that indebtedness will strongly influence physicians' values and alter their social contract to patients, with ethically deleterious consequences.

## 3. The rapid evolution of medical organizations

The new organizations buy up and/or otherwise regulate physicians' and other health practitioners' services via health maintenance organizations (HMOs), physician provider organizations (PPOs), independent provider associations (IPAs), and other managed care organizations. Within all of these entities forces operate that may constrain certain aspects of professional autonomy and decrease professionalism: deciding which tasks are to be performed by psychiatrists and which by other, less qualified, and less expensive mental health professionals such as "counselors"; setting physicians' standards for the pace and routine of work, the number of allotted visits, and for fees; and establishing bosses, such as insurance company case managers, to whom psychiatrists are accountable (Reed & Evans, 1987). Along with the regulation comes more paperwork—described as the "scut work of the 80's" (McCue, 1985, p. 450)—all of which reduces time with patients. In many aspects psychiatry is becoming less of a cottage industry than it used to be.

### 4. The supply of psychiatrists in the face of increasing competition with other providers

Official reports state that the nation needs more psychiatrists, and particularly more child psychiatrists, in contrast to most other medical specialties. However, in the face of rapidly changing demands due to economic retrenchment and increasing numbers of lower paid mental health professionals, the demand for services by psychiatrists for which someone will pay may be falling (Yager & Borus, 1987). However, there is still a great need for minority psychiatrists and for psychiatrists to work with currently underserved inner city and rural populations, areas which are unfortunately rife with stressors of their own. The roles of psychiatrists vis-à-vis other providers in the care of certain patient populations will be the subject of ongoing discussion, negotiation, debate, and controversy.

### 5. Changes in the knowledge base

The knowledge explosion taxes (but also enriches) psychiatry's practitioners. New knowledge assails us at so rapid a rate that few can even reasonably "keep up." As research has demonstrated, not only do physicians know what they don't know, they also *don't* know what they don't know (Williamson, German, & Weiss, 1989)! New technologies for learning and communication, such as videotape, interactive videodisc, online computers, and the soon-to-be-available videophone may be stressful in some respects; they will contribute even further to information overload, while causing some discomfort in those who haven't yet mastered the use of these instruments.

## Additional Stressors Affecting Psychiatrists in Executive Positions

With rapid expansion of the health industry in recent years and the escalation of costs, management has become the critical factor in an institution's survival. Management not only balances the budget, but sets the tone of an institution, and provides the proper conditions for treatment, training, and research. To a major degree, management influences the actual *level* of treatment success an institution enjoys.

In the last few decades there has been a radical shift in the leadership of mental institutions. As computerized information systems, regulatory agencies, and legal/judicial pronouncements regarding the treatment of patients have come forth, the task of the administrator has become more complicated and more stressful. Increasingly, professional administrators are replacing medical administrators. Professional managers, it should be noted, usually have received training in organizational dynamics, planning, budgeting, staff development, public relations, and law, among other areas. Some specifics regarding public sector psychiatric administrators will elucidate these issues.

Between 1971 and 1976, psychiatrists serving as directors of community mental health centers declined by 25% (Bass, 1979). In the state of New York, psychiatrists occupying senior administrative posts in the State Department of Mental Hygiene fell by 56% between 1975 and 1978 (Keill, 1978). Selection criteria clearly shifted away from medical knowledge to administrative ability and experience (Conway, 1982; Feldman, 1981).

During the period 1971–1981, the average length of service of state commissioners of mental health was 4.3 years, *excluding* acting commissioners and current commissioners; but the average length of stay *including* acting commissioners and *excluding* active commissioners was only 3.5 years (personal communication, Harry Schnibbe, Executive Director, National Association of State Mental Health Program Directors, 1983). At the same time, executives in mental health facilities indicate that it takes months to years before an incumbent feels accepted and competent (Strauss & Kohler, 1983). This means that the incumbent's period of confident and, hopefully, successful management is relatively short before they give way to an acting executive, whose terms average 0.8 years, or to a new appointee, who starts the learning process all over again. This process is obviously both illogical and wasteful. It signifies that during a large part of an incumbent's tenure, decision are really made by subordinates who survive through several successions, and who may, therefore, influence final decisions inordinately. During the short tenure, high mobilization of energies for rapid learning is required; and important decisions may be made without full comprehension of the consequences. Under these conditions, it is easy to understand that stressors acting upon the executive in charge may be very telling.

We have catalogued stressors and their consequent stressful impacts on psychiatrist in responsible executive posts in four studies (Gaver, Norman, & Greenblatt, 1984; Greenblatt, 1983; Greenblatt, Gaver, & Sherwood, 1985; Greenblatt & Rose, 1977). Altogether 147 respondents are represented; 109 of these were past commissioners of mental health, 30 were active (sitting) commissioners, and 8 were assorted executives: deans, hospital directors, or department chairmen.

We can summarize our research by saying that stressors and strains were *very* prominent experiences in the daily lives of these executives. Chief among these were work overload ("The job took more than 80 hours a week"); heavy responsibilities without adequate authority or resources; media and legislative pressures; strains on family life; frustrations in replacing incompetent staff with competent people; cumbersome institutional bureaucracies; and loneliness.

Based on our personal experience, we can add the following stressors to the list: lack of preparation for the job; high vulnerability to criticism, particularly as resources are not adequate to do a good job for all clients and families; political crossfires into which one is inevitably drawn as an appointee of a partisan governor; and an uncertain future. There is also the fact that, while on the job, the psychiatric executive moves further and further away from the center of their profession. If the executives come from an academic background, they may have the nagging feeling that they are too far away from students, teaching, and research. Furthermore, in the last decade there has been a progressive shift of power in institutions away from the clinician to the lay administrator. Thus the psychiatrist-executive finds himself or herself becoming an expert in a field that progressively abjures psychiatrists as legitimate members of the team. Finally, needless to say, the massive reduction in resources which characterizes the economy of so many institutions today has put an indelible stamp of tension on modern executive life.

# VULNERABILITY TO STRESSORS

Several factors are likely to contribute to the vulnerability of a given psychiatrist to the stressors which besiege them. For the most part, this vul-

nerability is likely to correlate with an absence of the many stress-protective factors discussed below. These factors may be considered as both
intrapersonal and interpersonal. Stated in the positive, protection against
vulnerability probably correlates with certain intrapersonal qualities of
temperament and personality such as resilience, hardiness, an optimistic
attitude, extroversion, and harm avoidance (Kobasa & Puccetti, 1983;
Maddi & Kobasa, 1984; Scheier, Weintraub, & Carver, 1985). Individuals
fortunately endowed with these temperamental characteristics may be
better able to find small daily pleasures rewarding to compensate for the
stressors they endure (Ornstein & Sobel, 1989). They operate by positively oriented, "up-beat" cognitions and axioms. Conversely, vulnerability to stressors is likely to be linked to a pessimistic outlook, tendencies
toward a depressive cognitive set, excessive stimulus seeking, introver-
sion, and neuroticism (Seligman, 1991). Those better able to be intraper-
sonally adaptive and flexible will be more likely to shift their practices,
learn and incorporate new paradigms in psychiatric theory, knowledge
and practice, and shift with the times. Translated to the interpersonal domain, such individuals will be better able to reach out for social and professional support and assistance for both practical and emotional needs as
they acquire new information, competencies, perspectives, and practice
patterns (Kobasa & Puccetti, 1983).

## COPING SKILLS AND PROTECTIVE FACTORS IN MANAGING STRESS

### General Physicians and General Psychiatrists

Studies regarding physician dissatisfaction with work reveal the most
commonly cited stressors to be heavy workload; on-call duties; lack of
personal free time; noncompliant and recalcitrant patients; dying patients
or patients not responding to treatment; interpersonal problems with
nurses and consultants; and excessive paperwork (Krakowski, 1982; Mawardi, 1979). Among recently graduated physicians, emerging stressors
included an increasing likelihood of malpractice suits; increasing reliance
on technology; violent attacks by angry patients; and concerns about
maintaining clinical competency (Mawardi, 1979).

A study we conducted of UCLA general physicians (Linn, Yager, Cope,
& Leake, 1985; Linn, Yager, Cope, and Leake, 1986a, 1986b) revealed
several important correlates of professional satisfaction that may help sug-

gest recommendations for enhancing professional satisfaction among psychiatrists as well. Compared to a general population sample of 1,297 who completed the same measure, both academic and community based physicians seemed equally or more satisfied with their jobs and their lives, rating themselves about 5.6 on a 7-point scale. The most commonly cited source of distress was time pressures—but we should point out that time pressure is also the most commonly cited source of distress by all other groups of professionals in our society—lawyers, businessmen, and accountants, for example. Difficult patients and other patient care issues were also cited as stressful, but were at the same time cited as sources of great satisfaction. This suggests that *stressors don't simply cause distress*. Overall, we found little to suggest that the physicians we studied worked longer hours, were more distressed, less satisfied, or in poorer health than other professional groups.

We also found that those physicians with more job satisfaction were more likely to use certain specific types of coping skills. First, job satisfaction was correlated with these physicians' attempts to organize and restructure their work activity—to take charge of their time. For example, 26% used special calendars and made lists daily, and 22% did so several times/week but about 22% never did. Thirty-nine percent blocked out time for making phone calls several times a week or daily; 63% reported specifically and routinely organizing and scheduling their work so they wouldn't be rushed or run late; 38% regularly reviewed their workload and reduced their expectations of what they could accomplish; and 15% attempted to restructure their practice by reorganizing or diversifying their activities on a regular basis. Other activities in this area included delegating work to others and cutting down on patient volume when feeling overloaded—practiced by about 45% of respondents. Physicians who expressed greater satisfaction with their work have somehow learned to manage their time more efficiently, are better organized, are more realistic regarding what they can accomplish, and are able to delegate responsibility and arrange and reorganize their workload frequently (Linn et al., 1986b).

General psychiatrists can cope with the stresses of their professional lives in a number of specific ways:

1. The first task for psychiatrists is to *situate themselves in practice eco-niches* that seem best fitted to their temperaments and inclinations. Practitioners must continually reflect on the extent to which they consider themselves to be generalists or subspecialists (Evans et al., 1989); biopsychosocialists or non-people-oriented technicians; continuity physicians or

short-term consultants; leaders or followers. Issues of pace, skill, and other important practical and emotional variables will influence the psychiatrist's choices regarding working hours, practice settings, practice arrangements, patient populations, and other aspects of professional life.

2. To cope with the explosion of knowledge, psychiatrists should *develop a systematic life-long learning plan* to continuously update their knowledge and skills based on their practice patterns; as with investing, systematic plans pay off. Each person may identify personal preferences and the most effective environments in which to keep reading and learning: e.g., home study, study groups, formal continuing education courses, and the like.

3. Psychiatrists need to *keep practicing critical thinking skills*, to better evaluate the strengths and weaknesses of the many sacred cows and new sacred calves that constantly appear—promoted by both academics and detail men.

4. Even those who are computerphobic should *learn the basics of computer use*. Hookups to *Grateful Med*, the National Library of Medicine's very inexpensive search software for home computers, which accesses MEDLINE and other databases, are simple to master and sources of endless, extremely current information. Computerphobia is easy to treat (Huth, 1989).

5. Even dedicated generalists can *enhance self-actualization by developing special expertise* in one or two specific clinical areas through mini-courses, practice, reading, and regular consultations. At the same time, psychiatrists should not become too devoted to a single technique or procedure, since the odds are great that it will be replaced by something new.

6. One can best satisfy needs for intellectual stimulation, creative growth, altruistic endeavour and autonomy by *setting up a schedule in which a certain amount of time is kept free*, religiously, for whatever aspects of psychiatry—or other interests—provide the greatest fulfillment. One should assume that the pleasure will pay very little or no money—such as volunteer teaching, serving the indigent, reading, or doing individual or collaborative creative scholarship or research. Generally speaking, active pastimes are more relaxing and satisfying than passive ones, and some physical activity is highly desirable in the busiest of professional schedules.

## Psychiatrist Administrators

Those in high administrative positions in psychiatry suffer from high rates of burnout and rapid turnover. Several studies have highlighted specific coping and protective factors in managing stress for these individuals, many of which factors may also serve general psychiatrists well:

## 1. Greater emphasis on preparation for the job.

As a group, many of the state mental health commissioners in our studies did not learn their work from formal sources, either coursework or books on administration (Greenblatt & Rose, 1977). Of the 109 former state mental health commissioners we studied in 1982–83, 14 said they had some training during residency; 21 in public health or university business school; and 14 had taken a fellowship oriented towards administration. In addition, many had had experience as superintendents or assistant superintendents of hospitals, some as Veterans Administration chiefs of service, and some as directors of public mental health clinics. The large majority of commissioners we polled (71.5%) did *not* have the American Psychiatric Association certificate in administration (Greenblatt et al., 1985).

More important, we think, than paper, pencil, or even oral examinations, would be the opportunity to learn from observation of and discussion with executives who have spent years in the saddle. Regular consultation and supervision would go far, we believe, to increase technical knowledge, promote perspective, and reduce stress. An astute senior supervisor could also do that all-important thing—point out how the executive himself played a role in the troubles he was in, as occurs in the supervision of psychotherapy.

## 2. Brief sabbaticals at selected or prescribed intervals.

Burnout is a hazard when problems multiply, health is impaired, or family problems complicate the executive's life. He should have a good deputy in whom he has confidence to take command in his absence, and he should be able to relinquish command when indicated. Time out and a less demanding schedule will permit reflection, reappraisal, and rejuvenation. At this juncture it may be wise to consult another administrator of experience or a wise therapist.

## 3. Cross visiting.

In cross-visiting, one executive spends time with another in a similar organization. The "visiting" executive can learn how generic his problems may be, and how they are solved elsewhere with, perhaps, less trouble. He develops friendships, shares feelings, solicits consultation, and advice.

Feelings of isolation and loneliness are reduced; and new perspectives emerge in relation to old ideas.

### Change in role and responsibility.

In many large institutions, personnel are moved from one unit to another, sometimes into the same level, sometimes higher, or even lower in the hierarchy. Although such moves may entail considerable uprooting, many executives accept this willingly as a reality of their career in the organization.

A change of role that is a promotion acts like a shot in the arm, but a new position, even at the same level, presents new challenges and new learning and permits freedom from old, tiring stressors.

### 5. Organizations and associations of administrators.

Several professional organizations of administrators meet regularly, provide for social and professional interchange, and encourage sharing of problems, and educational and research seminars. Among these may be listed:

American Association of Community Psychiatrists;
American Association of General Hospital Psychiatrists;
American College of Mental Health Administrators;
American Association of Chairmen of Departments of Psychiatry;
American Association of Directors of Psychiatric Residency Training; and
American Association of Veterans Affairs Chiefs of Staff;

Numerous exercises on administration are offered at annual meetings of these organizations and of the American Psychiatric Association. These include lectures, symposia, and workshops. At the annual APA Institute on Hospital and Community Psychiatry, professional meetings of nurses, social workers, occupational therapists, librarians, and administrators are also regularly scheduled.

### 6. Other sources of support.

To whom do state mental health commissioners turn for support? When the active commissioners were asked about their support systems, we learned that they felt most supported by hospital and clinic superintendents and directors, and least by the American Psychiatric Association. Community advisory groups and the National Association of State Mental Health Program Directors also gave substantial support. The negative feeling about the American Psychiatric Association is not surprising, since that organization has manifested little interest in state politics and paid no attention to the great loss of psychiatric leadership in state mental health organizations until recently.

### 7. Academic involvement.

Administrative jobs, however demanding, need not take the individual completely away from academe. Teaching appointments can be arranged in appropriate departments of schools and colleges, so that the individual can continue academic contact with their basic discipline. Both sides can only gain. The campus contact can stimulate student interest in administrative careers, and thus be an important recruiting tool in the search for future executives.

### 8. Subsequent careers.

Given the relatively short tenures of most state mental health commissioners, thoughts about "what next" may start on day one of the job. What prospects does the outgoing executive have for his or her future? Many psychiatric executives are concerned that time in office spent away from clinical practice, teaching, or research makes them "rusty" and thus less employable in desirable jobs in the field. It is often said that high-level administrative jobs are a dead end. This concept, together with limited tenure, the stresses and strains indicated above, lower financial return, and uncertain futures, are factors that make many shy away from executive responsibility.

## SATISFACTIONS AND REWARDS IN PSYCHIATRIC CAREERS

### General Psychiatrists

With all of the stressors delineated above, to what extent will the profession of psychiatry still be able to satisfy today's practitioners and administrators? Even with the shift in demographics among today's medical students and residents, the motivations of most contemporary trainees seem quite similar to those of the past. Most appear to have broad interests and are seeking challenging, stimulating, socially important, help-oriented, and prestigious careers that will concurrently provide a reasonable level of material comfort.

In examining the satisfactions that people seek from a medical career, Abraham Maslow's concepts of basic needs provide a useful framework (Maslow, 1954). Briefly, Maslow posited the existence of a hierarchy of needs, all of which must be satisfied if people are to achieve their full potential. At the most basic level are physiologic needs. The next level up consists of needs for safety and security: for protection, order, predictability, a sense of reality, and freedom from threat. Above these are social and affiliative needs: belonging, acceptance, affection, and group membership. Still further up in the hierarchy are needs for esteem, respect, and self-respect. At the top of the list are needs for self-actualization, activities that fulfill one's potential for autonomy, creativity, and altruistic effort.

According to Herzberg, Mausner, & Snyderman (1959), based on studies of various industries, people derive satisfaction from the nature of the work itself and from how well it meets their needs for achievement, recognition and respect. Work-related stressors and dissatisfaction stem primarily from concerns about basic security issues (e.g., safety), poor interpersonal relationships, and unpleasant policies, which presumably limit autonomy and self-control.

How do these various needs relate to today's careers in psychiatry? First, in spite of cost containment, it is likely that psychiatrists will continue to earn satisfactory incomes, on average higher than those of almost any other nonmedical profession or segment of the population. Of course, some people will not be satisfied, particularly when they contrast psychiatrists' with physicians' incomes of the past, and with the surgical specialties.

Regarding threat, safety, and security, such issues vary from practice to practice and hospital to hospital, and will continue to do so in the future. Unpleasant policies, an important contributor to work stressors and dissatisfaction, according to Herzberg et al. (1959), are of some concern and will be further discussed below.

With regard to a sense of reality, psychiatry offers a rich set of belief systems, most of increasing scientific validity, that ostensibly enable psychiatrists to make sense out of chaos and offer them some ability to better influence health, illness, and disease. These features are important stress reducers.

What about social and affiliative needs? In many ways, one of psychiatry's strongest attractions lies in its ability to satisfy affiliative needs. Many are attracted to the profession by fantasies involving the almost mystical psychiatrist-patient relationship, which they hope will provide some degree of *mutual* empathy, warmth and positive regard—encounters of true relatedness in an alienating world.

In addition to the gratifications of these clinical encounters, relationships with other health care providers and memberships in professional societies provide many social affiliations and a definite social role and identity. Professional opportunities for comradeship and a sharing of purpose and community occur through practice affiliations, faculty memberships, and participation in various professional societies.

The psychiatrist's needs for esteem, respect, and a sense of self-worth are met in several ways. First, the psychiatrist is viewed as a member of the generally well-regarded medical profession, a "learned profession", usually seen as necessary and helpful; enabled to share humanistic and theoretically altruistic values that most people find admirable; able to achieve professional goals and obtain positive feedback from patients and others; and, of course, able to develop a sense of professional competence through skillful helping, fixing, curing, and improving—reducing stress through a sense of personal effectiveness.

Finally, psychiatry provides, and will continue to provide, more potential avenues for self-actualization than most other professions: the chance to master clinical challenges and technical procedures; to artfully combine science and intuition; to continuously grow and learn; to autonomously make decisions and act on them; to constantly make choices regarding professional activities, special interest areas, time allocation, and work-setting; to engage in scientific discovery and intellectual creativity; and to behave altruistically. All of these features contribute to personal satisfaction and help to combat personal distress.

## Additional Satisfactions and Rewards for Psychiatrist Administrators

Psychiatry administration offers its own special set of circumstances and rewards, spanning across the Maslowian hierarchy. Today's psychiatrists have to accept the fact that management is an inescapable part of medical life. One is either a manager or a managee, and usually some of both. Psychiatrists must decide for themselves how much they want to be part of management; how much management they're willing to delegate—or abdicate—to someone else in order to spend time doing other things; and what they're willing to give up for either choice. Regardless of how much or how little administration one does, the challenge is to become involved constructively in the management of one's various work organizations, professional societies, and with the larger societal context in which they operate; and to maximize one's input regarding goals and quality of services to patients and to professional satisfaction. Since "unpleasant policies" are great sources of stressors and job dissatisfaction, administration is the place that one can at least attempt to do something about them.

Some are attracted to leadership roles by virtue of temperament and talents, and others find themselves reluctantly and unwillingly drawn into such roles by situational demands to which no one else responds. These roles occur in many contexts and at many levels—from the unit chief to the chief executive officer of a private psychiatric corporation, and from the crisis service or aftercare director of a mental health center to the state commissioner for mental health. These roles vary considerably in the responsibility, authority, autonomy, accountability, and resources that they carry.

Although the stressors acting on the executive are severe, the rewards can be exhilarating. Again, summarizing the results of several studies, executives stressed the rewards of contributing significantly to the field of mental health, building programs, and making a difference in health care delivery and education (Gaver et al., 1984; Greenblatt, 1983; Greenblatt et al., 1985; Greenblatt & Rose, 1977). Frequent references were made to personal growth, increase in self-confidence, and the joy of facing and overcoming major challenges. New personal relationships with interesting and important persons were rewarding. Prestige and recognition were things to enjoy, as was the feeling of power, not just power in the ego-expansive sense, but power to control affairs and to do good for many. Some state mental health commissioners have found a gratifying role in protecting the values of professionals serving the mentally ill, for in the course of the scrambles that take place in the arena, professional ideals of service may be attacked, or attempts made to limit the freedom to do research; or legislation may be introduced to shape professional education.

In addition, the 109 ex-state mental health commissioners queried in this regard reported a high level of satisfaction with jobs obtained post-commissionership, including jobs in public and private administration (Greenblatt et al., 1985). Although desired academic jobs were obtained less often than nonacademic jobs, the overall rate of wish-fulfillment was 84%. The concern that high-level executive experience will not be valued in the marketplace would seem to be invalid. As might be expected, our data also revealed that where subsequent job satisfaction was high (i.e., with the job *after* commissioner), few former commissioners were willing to serve again as commissioner. Contrariwise, where subject job satisfaction was low, more subjects evinced a willingness to serve as commissioner again.

We found a strong negative relationship between level of satisfaction with jobs after commissionership and a phenomenon we identified as "decompression" (Greenblatt et al., 1985). "Decompression" was defined as a sudden decrease in work intensity, centrality in the action scene, power, and public visibility, such as accompanied a sudden shift from a high-level responsibility to a low-level job responsibility. Decompression seemed to us to be a special case of depression in a specific psychosocial context. It was different from "burnout," the term usually applied to the person who becomes jaded, bored, and depressed in a busy and demanding job. Subjects who reported much decompression were less satisfied with subsequent jobs, and often were willing to serve again as commissioners. They felt that a great deal had been left unfinished in the previous job.

## CONCLUSION

Although the stressors acting on practicing psychiatrists and psychiatric administrators in particular are increasingly complex, we can nevertheless anticipate that their basic professional needs for safety and security, affiliation, esteem, and self-actualization can be well satisfied within the practice and administrative climates envisioned in the near future. Among the many stress-protective and vulnerability reducing factors for the profession, we can anticipate increasingly powerful psychiatric treatments that will further enhance the mystique of psychiatry and increase the public's respect for the profession. Psychiatric practitioners and psychiatric administrators should familiarize themselves with and take advantage of all available coping skills and support systems that afford additional protection from stress. For the practitioner, these include professional affiliations and active participation in professional organizations, maintaining and enhancing professional competence through ongoing personal development in general psychiatry and in areas of special subspecialty interest, engaging in scientific and intellectual creativity and scholarship, effective use of time management techniques that assures discretionary time for areas of special professional or non-professional interests, and altruistic professional activities. For the psychiatric administrator these include adequate preparation for their jobs, brief sabbaticals to reduce burnout, cross-visiting with other administrators and institutions, shifting roles and responsibilities, academic involvement, and participation in professional organizations for psychiatric administrators.

Each individual needs to identify the types and levels of their need and to honestly assess their own abilities to be tough, take criticism, roll with the punches, and enjoy the challenges, before deciding on the specific career line to follow. For all of the many stresses imposed by careers in general psychiatry and in psychiatric administration, we envision that those fortunate enough to find themselves in such careers will continue to enjoy ample opportunities for making meaningful contributions to the care of suffering patients and for achieving satisfying and rewarding professional lives.

# REFERENCES

Bass, R. D. (1979). *CMHC staffing: Who minds the store?* Rockville, MD: National Institute of Mental Health.

Conway, A. (1982). Psychiatric management: Change in the 1980s. *Hospital and Community Psychiatry, 33*, 310–311.

Evans, R. G., Lomas, J., Barer, M. L., Labelle, R. J., Fooks, C., Stoddart, G. S., Anderson, G. M., Feeny, D., Gafni, A., & Torrance, G. W. (1989). Controlling health expenditures: The Canadian Reality. *New England Journal of Medicine, 320*, 571–577.

Feldman, S. (1981). Leadership in mental health: Changing the guard for the 1980s. *American Journal of Psychiatry, 138*, 1147–1153.

Gaver, K. D., Norman, M. L., & Greenblatt, M. (1984). Life at the state summit: Views and experiences of 18 psychiatric leaders. *Hospital and Community Psychiatry, 35*, 233–238.

Greenblatt, M. (1983). Management succession: Some major parameters. *Administration in Mental Health, 11*, 3–10.

Greenblatt, M., Gaver, K. D., & Sherwood, E. (1985). After commissioner, what? *American Journal of Psychiatry, 6*, 752–754.

Greenblatt, M., & Rose, S. O. (1977). Illustrious psychiatric administrators. *American Journal of Psychiatry, 134*, 626–630.

Herzberg, F., Mausner, B., & Snyderman, B. (1959). *The motivation to work.* New York: Wiley.

Huth, E. J. (1989). The underused medical literature. *Annals of Internal Medicine, 110*, 99–100.

Keill, S. L. (1978). Psychiatrists and state mental health systems. *Psychiatric Opinion, 15*, 10–16.

Kobasa, S. C., & Puccetti, M. C. (1983). Personality and social resources in stress-resistance. *Journal of Personality and Social Psychology, 45*, 839–50.

Krakowski, A. (1982). Stress and the Practice of medicine: II. Stressors, stresses and strains. *Psychotherapy and Psychosomatics, 38*, 11–23.

Linn, L. S., Yager, J., Cope, D., & Leake, B. (1985). Health status job satisfaction, job stress, and life satisfaction among academic and clinical faculty. *Journal of the American Medical Association, 254*, 2775–2782.

Linn, L. S., Yager, J., Cope, D., & Leake, B. (1986a). Health habits and coping behaviors among practicing physicians. *Western Journal of Medicine, 144*, 484–489.

Linn, L. S., Yager, J., Cope, D., & Leake, B. (1986b). Factors associated with life satisfaction among practicing physicians. *Medical Care, 24*, 830–837.

Maddi, S. R., & Kobasa, S. C. (1984). *The hardy executive: Health under stress.* Homewood, IL: Dow Jones-Irwin.

Maslow, A. (1954). *Motivation and personality.* New York: Harper and Row.

Mawardi, B. H. (1979). Satisfactions, dissatisfactions and causes of stress in medical stress. *Journal of the American Medical Association, 241*, 1483–1486.

McCue, J. D. (1985). The distress of internship: Causes and prevention. *New England Journal of Medicine, 312*, 449–451.

Ornstein, R., & Sobel, D. (1989). *Healthy pleasures.* Reading, MA: Addison-Wesley.

Oryshkevich, B. A. (1989). [Letter to the editor]. *New England Journal of Medicine, 320*, 188.

Rabkin, M. T. (1982). The SAG Index. *New England Journal of Medicine, 307*, 1350–1351.

Reed, R. R., & Evans, D. (1987). The deprofessionalism of medicine: Causes, effects and responses. *Journal of the American Medical Association, 258*, 3279–3282.

Scheier, M. F., Weintraub, J. K., & Carver, C. S. (1986). Coping with stress: Divergent strategies of optimists and pessimists. *Journal of Personality and Social Psychology, 51*, 1257–64.

Schnibbe, H. (1983). Executive Director, National Association of State Mental Health Program, personal communication.

Seligman, M. E. P. (1991). *Learned optimism.* New York: Knopf.

Shiao, W. C., Braun, P., Dunn, D., Becker, E. R., De Nicola, M., & Ketchan, T. R. (1988). Results and policy implications of the resource based relative-value study. *New England Journal of Medicine, 319*, 881–888.

Strauss, G. D., & Kohler, T. (1983). Executive succession in health care organizations. *Administration in Mental Health, 11*, 22–35.

Weismann, Sidney H. (in press). Recommendations from the May 1992 Conference on Recruitment of United States Medical Graduates into Psychiatry. *Academic Psychiatry.*

Williamson, J. W., German, P. S., & Weiss, R. (1989). Health science information management and continuing education of physicians. *Annals of Internal Medicine, 110*, 151–160.

Yager, J., & Borus, J. F. (1987). Are we training too many psychiatrists? *American Journal of Psychiatry, 144*, 1172–1177.

# Index

# A

Abdominal distension, 26
Acetylcholine, function of, 9
Achievement Center, 72
Acoma-Caanoncito-Laguna Teen
    Center, 111
Acquired skills
    durability, 63–64
    generalizability, 64–66
ACTH
    depression and, 38, 44
    electric shock and, 14
    levels of, 10
    major depression and, 43
    reaction suppression, 7
    secretion of, 18
Acute combat reaction
    precipitants, 87–88
    prevention of, 89–90
    signs and symptoms, 84, 86, 88
    treatment of, 88–89
Acute stress, long-term conse-
    quences of, 12–14
Adenylate cyclase, 16
Adjustment disorders, Indian/Native
    American youth, 105
Adjuvant arthritis, 20–21
Adrenal cortex, 44
Adrenal medullary hormones, 40
Adrenalectomy, 7, 14
Affective disorders, Indian/Native
    American youth, 105

Aftercare programs, 73
Alarm reaction, 39
Alcohol abuse, 55, 107
Alien Tort Claims Act (1979), 131
Allergic reaction, 7
American Association of Chairmen
    of Departments of Psychiatry,
    170
American Association of Commu-
    nity Mental Health Psychia-
    trists, 170
American Association of Directors of
    Psychiatric Residency Training,
    170
American Association of General
    Hospital Psychiatrists, 170
American Association of Veterans
    Affairs Chief of Staff,
    170
American College of Mental Health
    Administrators, 170
American Psychiatric Association,
    170–171
Amnesty International, 142–143
Anabolic hormones, 40
Androgenic metabolites, 40
Anesthesia, stress research and, 3
Animal isolation, stress research and,
    3
Anorexia nervosa, 18
Anticipatory phase, response pat-
    tern, 9–10

181